Praise for *Wall of Silence*

"Gibson and Singh provide a call to arms for families who have had loved ones disabled or die in the pursuit of medical treatment. . . . Well written and researched, [*Wall of Silence*] highlights this timely topic in a unique way that will evoke the reader's own experiences." **—Former First Lady Rosalynn Carter**

"The tragic accounts gathered here . . . are a warning. They remind us of the importance of being careful and alert, whatever we do, of the need to help wherever we can, and, where we cannot, at least to prevent harm. Real care of the sick does not begin with costly procedures, but with the cultivation of a kind heart."
—His Holiness the Dalai Lama

"Every patient needs to read this book."
—Ellen Stovall, Executive Director,
National Coalition for Cancer Survivorship

"Exciting! Tremendous that *Wall of Silence* has been written. The horror stories have to be told."
—James E. Burke, Former Chairman
and CEO, Johnson & Johnson

"Timely and extraordinary. . . The authors portray riveting stories of medical errors and what needs to be done to solve this vexing problem. A must-read for patients and families on how they can protect themselves."
—The Honorable Thomas Kean,
Former Governor, State of New Jersey

"*Wall of Silence* does something no one else has done—tell the real stories of medical errors."

"In a clear and eloquent voice, *Wall of Silence* reinforces an issue that the health care system has not wanted to address."

"*Wall of Silence* does a really terrific job of putting a face on the statistics regarding medical error. . . . [D]emonstrates many of the different ways this serious problem is manifest throughout the health care system."

"This very readable and comprehensive book puts medical errors in a compelling human context. The lay reader will better understand the complex underlying issues that affect mistakes being made, but also will better understand the human toll."

"*Wall of Silence* should be required reading for every American who uses, or is a potential user of, the health care system. . . . [W]ithout placing unfair blame on dedicated health providers, the authors alert us to this major and complex problem. Most important, it empowers each of us to guard against being a victim by being an educated consumer. . . . Wall of Silence will serve as a wake-up call for each of us."

"...a repository of information and a set of clear opportunities for safety that the public can use."

—*Geraldine Bednash, R.N., Ph.D., F.A.A.N., Executive Director, American Association of Colleges of Nursing*

"This is a book that should interest all Americans, as we are all affected by the health care system. With an array of examples that are revealing and sometimes shocking, the authors clearly illustrate many of the systemic problems that need addressing and offer some pragmatic steps that the public and health care professionals can take to enhance the reliability of care.

—*The Honorable Matthew F. McHugh, Former Congressman from New York*

"A compelling story of what the public needs to be concerned about."

—*William Roper, M.D., M.P.H., Dean, School of Public Health, University of North Carolina at Chapel Hill, Former Director, Centers for Disease Control Former Administrator, Health Care Financing Administration Former White House health care advisor*

"Gibson and Singh have moved beyond statistics, or 'system' terminology, to put the human face, and story, in front of us. Nurses, doctors, pharmacists, patients, and families want care to be safer, and *Wall of Silence* illustrates how that can be done."

—*Mary Foley, M.S., R.N., Past President, American Nurses Association*

"The harrowing stories by patients and their families—and physicians—reveal an urgent need for sweeping changes in the culture of medicine. Gibson and Singh speak to the necessary review of physicians' efforts toward patient care."

—Eric J. Hodgson, M.D., National President 2002–2003,
American Medical Student Association

"I'm so happy that Gibson and Singh have given voice to those of us who have suffered at the hands of this broken and greed-driven health care industry."

—Kay McVay, R.N., President, California Nurses Association

wallofsilence

wallofsilence

The Untold Story of the
Medical Mistakes That Kill
and Injure Millions of Americans

Rosemary Gibson
and
Janardan Prasad Singh

LifeLine
Press®

A Regnery Publishing Company
Washington, D.C.

Library of Congress Cataloging-in-Publication Data on file.

ISBN 0-89526-112-X

Published in the United States by

LifeLine Press

A Regnery Publishing Company

One Massachusetts Avenue, N.W.

Washington, DC 20001

Visit us at www.lifelinepress.com

Distributed to the trade by

National Book Network

4720-A Boston Way

Lanham, MD 20706

Printed on acid-free paper

Manufactured in the United States of America

10 9 8 7 6 5 4 3

Books are available in quantity for promotional or premium use. Write to Director of Special Sales, Regnery Publishing, Inc., One Massachusetts Avenue, N.W., Washington, DC 20001, for information on discounts and terms or call (202) 216-0600.

The stories in this book are true, related to the authors by real people. They are not composites, nor have details such as gender, age, or medical error been altered. In some instances people's names have been changed at their request, to protect their identity and maintain their privacy.

To those who shared their stories
and to those whose stories remain untold

Content

Acknowledgments

This book would not have been possible without the courage and determination of the people who graciously shared their experiences with medical error that changed them forever. There are no words to express our heartfelt appreciation to them for allowing us into their lives in the aftermath of error, in all its anguish and devastation. If we have accomplished nothing else with this book, we hope it gives voice to the silent suffering they and many others have sustained. Our fervent wish is that we have done justice to their sorrow and their hope for a better tomorrow.

We are grateful to Ilene Corina and Jennifer Dingman, who introduced us to the vast network of people all across America who have borne the consequences of medical mistakes. Lennie and Ed Duensing shared their enthusiasm, hospitality, and encouragement while we wrote this book. For his unerring faith in this endeavor from the very beginning, we are indebted to Gail Warden. Those who patiently waded through various drafts have our heartfelt thanks—Bernice Harper, Booker Woods, Larry and Lois Jassie, Yiota Souras, Jean Johnson, Ranjan Dwivedi, Nisha Singh, and Sarveshwari Singh. Joseph Alper helped turn an early draft into compelling narrative. Kathy Flatley and Mary Beth Kren shared the fruit of their expertise as searchers of valuable information. Susan

Leisentritt made scraps of paper into something readable with precision and care.

Marji Ross, Molly Mullen, and Mike Ward at LifeLine Press understood the importance and timeliness of the message of this book, and we shall remain ever grateful to them. They had faith in this work and wisely encouraged us to put a human face on a profound national problem that deserves urgent resolve and resolution.

Finally, we render our humble and profoundest regard to the one who inspired this book and who has made it—and so much else—possible.

Preface

For several years, we cared for a beloved friend who had a life-threatening medical condition. He received the best care the U.S. health system had to offer. It prolonged his life, and we are profoundly and eternally grateful to the many doctors, nurses, and others who cared for him. But what the health care system gave with one hand, it took away with the other. He died because of medical error.

During one of his many hospitalizations, a nurse came into his room to administer his usual dose of medication. As she poured his medicine, she filled the cup with almost three times the usual dose of a very powerful drug. We were standing by the bed, and one of us exclaimed, "That seems to be a lot more than what he usually takes." The nurse reread the prescription order—which was nearly illegible, realized the mistake, and reduced the dose she gave him. With the exhausted look that comes with finishing a double shift and taking care of many other very sick patients, she thanked us profusely and left the room.

A few weeks later, we asked his doctor what would happen if too much of the drug were ingested by mistake, without saying anything about the near miss. He said it could cause serious complications and possibly lead to death. It was pure chance, or even providence, that we were present and vigilant at the very moment when the life that we had worked so hard to sustain could have started on a downward spiral toward death.

But eventually it did. A string of other errors were too much for his body to bear. Doctors streamed in and out of the revolving door, but no one was in charge. No matter what we did, no matter how many days and nights we spent at bedside vigil, it was no match for the giant careless machine that extinguished the life we cherished more than our own.

Several years after this devastating loss, a committee of some of the nation's preeminent health care leaders, assembled by the prestigious Institute of Medicine of the National Academy of Sciences, issued a report whose findings were startling. Nearly 100,000 Americans die every year from medical errors, and thousands more are injured and disabled. This is almost the number of deaths from breast cancer, AIDS, and traffic accidents combined. We came to realize that the errors we had witnessed several years before were not a rare event. Rather, they were very common.

All along, unbeknown to us, a flame was burning inside, stoked by the growing clamor about people who have died or been injured by the "care" in health care. Looking back, we never thought of what we had witnessed as "error" or "mistake." But so it was. Now there was a language to name the real cause of death. The next step was to put a human face on these preventable tragedies.

We wrote this book to show that there are real people behind the national statistics and to tell their stories. At first, we thought it would be hard to find other people affected by medical errors. To the contrary, it wasn't hard at all. We discovered networks of people who have been harmed, and support groups cropping up all over the country. Who are these people coming forward to tell their stories? They make the cars we drive, patrol our streets, raise the cows that produce the milk we drink, tell us about the day's news on network television, and guard the security of our country from the White House and the field. Some of them are their children. Others are their parents. From all walks of life, they come. And they keep coming.

As we were writing the book and mentioned the topic to friends, neighbors, and coworkers, we discovered that many of them had a story they were eager to tell. Some had been prescribed drugs when their medical condition would warrant them never to be prescribed. Others told tales of poorly performed surgeries that caused so much pain that their loved ones lost the will to live. In one instance, only a second surgery by a competent orthopedist fixed a failed surgery; fortunately the pain receded and the patient recovered. Breakdowns in communication among health professionals were pervasive and put people at risk. Especially striking were the stories told by doctors, nurses, and health care administrators whose own loved ones suffered the effects of medical mistakes. No one is immune.

Those who bear the consequences of medical mistakes—and their families—carry a burden that is in no way reflected in the grim statistics. For some, a part of who they are is literally gone as a result of surgical or other mistakes. For others, their families have only memories of a loved one, and the ache in the heart of survivors is palpable. The rage is like a rising tide ready to wash away everything in its wake.

Fear reigns among those who have vowed to stay as far away as possible from a system that harms. Some are resigned to the inevitability. Many have no choice but to go back to the place where they've been harmed; they have no money to go anywhere else. Others don't want to think about it.

Meanwhile, the view from the other side of the bedrails is sobering. Doctors and nurses describe the imposed silence that shrouds medical mistakes. Fearful of lawsuits, hospitals encourage these doctors and nurses to keep silent about medical mistakes they are involved in or observe. The paralyzing fear of making a mistake, and hurting someone whom they intend to heal, is profound. They bemoan the chaos in many health care settings where they work, conditions that are breeding grounds for mistakes. Then there are the stories of some of their peers who are incompetent and who should not retain the privilege of caring for patients. And there are the tragedies that ensue when the medical profession covers up untold harm and fails to expel those members they would never want caring for themselves or their loved ones.

We will introduce you to some of the people who live in the aftermath of medical mistakes and whose stories are not easy to read. They are stories of courageous people speaking out with the intent to expose the underbelly of our health care system. And they hope that others like them will know they are not alone and derive strength from their courage.

An enlightened hospital CEO said, "Putting a human face on medical mistakes can increase the pressure to do something about them." That's another reason we wrote this book. We hope that the many faces of medical mistakes, coming out from behind the wall of silence, will make the stakes of the health system doing nothing much too high for the public to bear.

Deaths and injuries from errors occur not from the natural course of disease or injury, but from the care provided. They are preventable. More often than not, errors occur because health care is poorly organized and hospitals are understaffed; a string of small failures adds up to cause the greatest heartbreak and the most tragic results. They also occur because doctors and hospitals are doing procedures and tests they don't know how to do well, and still get paid for them.

Our greatest hope is that this book will save lives. With more awareness about how the system itself causes preventable harm, the public will know they need to be vigilant. But as from our own experience, vigilance goes only so far.

Our greatest yearning is for CEOs of hospitals, members of boards of trustees of health care organizations, and other medical and industry leaders to look within to see how many preventable deaths and injuries are occurring on their watch, and be motivated to make them as rare as possible.

The biggest mistake is the failure to act in the face of preventable injury and death. The health care industry is a laggard behind virtually all other sectors of our economy in allowing unsafe service to proliferate. This is the most egregious error of them all.

Finally, you will hear how the health system treats people in the aftermath of a medical mistake. If the reader thinks that errors are bad enough, it may be surprising to learn that the aftermath, and how people are treated, can be as painful as the error itself. The plea from patients and families who have been harmed is that mistakes need to be disclosed, apologies must be rendered, and amends made.

Many of the people you will meet in this book have been unsuccessful in getting the health care system to acknowledge and be accountable for errors that changed their lives forever. So they are channeling their anguish and anger into advocacy for reform. Some are too ill or in too much physical pain to speak out; others have been beaten down by the system. Those who fight for health care that does no harm are motivated by the desire to prevent the same mistake from happening to someone else. Without an organized political constituency—at least not yet, the battle is a lonely one. More often than not, the system quashes the truth they speak and the accountability they seek.

They have a lot in common with conscientious providers of health care who no longer want to bear witness to the suffering. Many of them are victims, too, of a system where mistakes are waiting to happen. From both sides of the bedrails, much more unites than divides. We hope this book will spur a united front to make health care accountable for what it gets paid to do.

All of us—patients, families, doctors, nurses, pharmacists, hospital administrators, civic leaders, employers, senior citizens, members of the media, and elected officials—have a stake in the outcome. The reason is that any one of us could be next.

Rosemary Gibson
Janardan Prasad Singh
April 2003

part one

Breaking the Silence

1 | Shattering Losses

Ilene and George's son Michael should be a teenager now. He should be getting ready to take the SATs and choosing the colleges to which he wants to apply. His parents, both postal workers on Long Island, wish they were grappling with how they'll manage the cost of college tuition. The teenager might be following in his dad's footsteps and thinking about how a promising record on the high school baseball team could give him an edge to receive a college scholarship.

Instead, a park in North Wantagh, Long Island, has a playground dedicated in his name. Michael suffered the effects of a medical mistake that turned a routine surgical procedure into a death knell for a three-year-old boy.

Michael Louis was born July 8, 1987, Ilene and George's first child. Brown-eyed, with huge dimples, he enjoyed playing with the other children at his baby sitter's house. Soon after his first birthday, the start of what would become chronic ear infections began, and he became a regular visitor to his pediatrician's office. Antibiotics would knock down his infection, but his tonsils and adenoids were large. By the time he was two and a half, they had grown so large that his pediatrician recommended that Michael's tonsils and adenoids be removed.

In the 1960s and 1970s, many children had their tonsils removed. Today, doctors perform 80 percent fewer tonsillectomies on children than they did in 1970. Medical research has shown that removing a child's tonsils and adenoids may not be very effective in helping children whose sore throat infections don't meet certain standards of frequency and severity, and the benefits don't outweigh the risks. Michael's parents were aware of the risks, but after visiting a surgeon and obtaining medical opinions from two additional doctors, the couple decided to go ahead with the operation.

On the morning of Tuesday, March 6, 1990, a surgeon removed Michael's tonsils and adenoids at a hospital in New York. He went home later that day, and his doctor told his parents to watch him carefully for any signs of bleeding, which occurs in a small percentage of children who have their tonsils removed.

The next day, Michael seemed to be well on the way to recovery, but the following morning, Thursday, Ilene noticed blood on her son's pillow. She called the surgeon's office immediately and was told to bring him in so he could be examined. There, the doctor cauterized, or sealed, the leaking blood vessels around the surgery wound. Two days later, Ilene again noticed blood in her son's teeth, and soon after waking he began vomiting blood and blood clots. Ilene called the emergency room, and the nurse answering the phone peppered her with questions while telling her that this wasn't an emergency—if it was, she would have told Ilene to call 911.

But while Ilene was on the phone, the boy threw up blood again, so she hung up on the nurse, put him in her car, and sped to the hospital. "If only I'd called nine-one-one, Michael might be alive," Ilene recounted recently.

Up to this point, there's little fault to find with the way the medical system responded to the postoperative problems. Michael's surgeon did as practice demands by cauterizing the vessels that were the source of the boy's bleeding. The emergency room nurse responded correctly, trying to ease Ilene's fears. To be sure, the tod-

dler was a statistic, one of the small number of children who suffer bleeding after having their tonsils and adenoids removed. But
when mother and son came through the emergency room doors,
Ilene's dark-blue sweatshirt caked with blood, the medical system
began to fail.

The emergency room staff took Michael's vital signs—his blood
pressure and temperature were both low, signs of shock that were
ignored. The staff advised Ilene to take him to see the surgeon.
Unfortunately, the surgeon couldn't be reached that day, and a
pediatrician from the same clinic, a stranger to the family, dismissed her concerns and sent them home. Later, Ilene remembers
thinking that if she'd been wearing white instead of blue, perhaps
they would have taken her concerns more seriously. "I had so
much blood on my sweatshirt, it looked like I had been a gunshot
victim," she said.

The next day, the toddler's groin was terribly swollen, and
welts—big open sores—covered his bottom. Ilene once again took
her son into the clinic. On duty that day was an allergist who had
seen Michael for an unrelated problem; he prescribed an ointment
for the sores and mother and son went home once again.

Tuesday was the day of the one-week follow-up appointment
with the surgeon, who was surprised at the boy's condition. He
told Ilene that he had not been informed of the weekend's events,
but he didn't seem concerned. No blood work was ordered and no
blood pressure or temperature readings were taken. The boy just
needed to avoid solid food for a few more days.

On Wednesday, Ilene took her son to the baby sitter's house so
she could return to work at the post office after having taken the
previous week off to care for her son. Not long afterward, the boy
began throwing up large amounts of blood, and in a panic, the
baby sitter called Ilene at work and then called 911. Ilene rushed
to the baby sitter's home, finding her son limp and unresponsive,
blood soaking the carpeting in the baby sitter's living room. A
policeman gently took the boy from Ilene's arms to bring him out

to the ambulance—it was the last time she held her son alive. Michael Louis died of blood loss that Wednesday, soon after reaching the hospital. A review of the boy's care found that from his first visit to the emergency room, the health care system had failed the little boy. A physician wrote, "It is my opinion, based upon a reasonable degree of medical certainty, that a significant and unusual postoperative history was ignored. The failure to make any determination on just how much blood this child had lost allowed him to persist in a precarious state whereby the next bleed was likely to be fatal."

On March 14, 1990, just a week after a routine procedure, Michael had become one of the tens of thousands of people, young and old, who suffer needless deaths each year resulting from preventable medical mistakes. Michael's death devastated his parents. His dad would get dressed for work and leave the house but never show up for work. Ilene discovered this only after a chance meeting with his manager. Struggling to keep herself healthy, she had to find a way to give her husband a reason to keep on living. They joined a support group for parents of deceased children, but their son's death was different from all others. It wasn't from a disease or injury. The ripples of devastation went beyond Michael's parents. His grandparents, aunts and uncles, friends and neighbors, even the policemen who responded to the 911 call, realized someone very special had been lost forever.

So Much Harm, So Little Done

Many Americans have their own story to tell about medical care that went awry because of mistakes that didn't have to happen. They are stories of people from all walks of life. As one woman whose father suffered the effects of a medical mistake wrote to us in an e-mail, "It happened to me, it could happen to you. It happens to the old, the young, the rich, the poor, the educated, the uneducated." She's right. Here are just a few:

• a World War II Army veteran and member of the greatest generation who served his country and had a zest for life as a professional golfer, yet who died of a medical mistake after surgery;

• a former White House official whose daily excruciating pain after a botched surgery has left a brilliant man in the prime of his life a virtual prisoner in his own home, unable to work;

• an Emmy award-winning television news anchor who lost just about everything because of a cosmetic procedure that went terribly awry;

• an Air Force intelligence officer whose care after hip replacement surgery was so bad that it has taken years of follow-up surgeries to repair the damage;

• an eight-year-old girl who—despite the misdiagnosed cancer that has left her paralyzed—has forgiven the doctors who missed the cancer and worries about how bad they must feel;

• a ninety-four-year-old grandmother in Florida, still an active hospital volunteer even at that age, who climbed over a hospital bed railing following a routine surgical procedure after her cries to go to the bathroom were ignored. She fell, breaking her hip, and died from complications related to the surgery needed to repair the fracture.

Medical mistakes don't always lead to death or injury. Sometimes they can cause unnerving fear. The *Detroit News* told of a sixty-six-year-old Michigan woman who went to the hospital to have a kidney stone removed. After she returned home, the hospital called her with devastating news. The instruments used to remove the kidney stone may not have been sterilized properly before they were used. As a result, she and twenty other patients may have been exposed to HIV, the virus that causes AIDS, and other infectious microbes. She now needs to be tested every six weeks for the rest of her life to make sure she has not contracted AIDS or any other diseases. She finds it hard to fathom how a hospital procedure exposed her to such risk. As she said to the *Detroit News* about the hospital, "They're in the business of making you healthy, not sick."[1]

And then there are the near misses, the mistakes that could have happened, but were caught in time. A father told the story of his five-year-old daughter, who had a successful bone marrow transplant, a state-of-the-art therapy for cancer.[2] After the procedure, she was transferred to the pediatric floor in the hospital. Her parents stayed overnight in her room and tried to remain awake so they could check the drugs that the nurses came to administer. One night shortly before the girl was to go home, her mother opened her eyes to find a nurse preparing to put something into her daughter's intravenous line. She asked the nurse what it was, and the nurse replied that it was what the doctor ordered. The mother insisted on knowing what the medication was, so she got up, read the order, and checked the drug. It was the right drug and the right dose, but it was meant for another patient. This is just one of several preventable and life-threatening mistakes that occurred during this little girl's brave fight against cancer. She lost the battle shortly before her sixth birthday.

The problem of medical mistakes is not just the sum of all the human tragedies that lie in their wake. Medical mistakes highlight a peculiar characteristic of our health care system, namely that so much harm is done to so many people, yet so little is done to publicly acknowledge and report preventable deaths and to disclose to patients and their families that a devastating outcome was preventable. No comfort or support is rendered to those who suffer great loss. This is the underlying story—and the real tragedy—of medical mistakes.

Stunning Rates of Medical Errors

In the fall of 1999, nearly a decade after young Michael bled to death following the tonsillectomy, a distinguished group of leaders in American health care, working under the auspices of the Institute of Medicine (IOM) of the National Academy of Sciences, reported that as many as 98,000 people in the United States die each year from medical mistakes in hospitals—mistakes that could be prevented.[3] The report also noted that tens of thousands more suffer permanent injuries as a result of such errors, and billions of dollars are spent treating the injuries.

From the time Michael died to the time the IOM published its startling report, nearly a million people may have died not innocently from disease or injury but as victims of medical mistakes that occurred during the care they received for their illness or injury. William Richardson, the chair of the committee that prepared the report, said, "These stunningly high rates of medical errors—resulting in deaths, permanent disability, and unnecessary suffering—are simply unacceptable in a medical system that first promises to 'do no harm.'"

Actually, the staggering number of medical mistakes was not a new finding. Eight years earlier, the *New England Journal of Medicine*, one of the most highly regarded and widely read medical journals in the world, published the research findings that helped to serve as the basis for the IOM estimates.[4] But in 1991 there was little if any outcry or comment about these findings. No governments enacted laws to protect patients and their families. The medical profession and health care organizations carried on, business as usual.

Thirty million Americans step into the scary and unfamiliar world of a hospital every year and put their trust and their lives in the hands of doctors, nurses, and administrators. It seems reasonable to expect that somebody would have done something to prevent medical mistakes from occurring. It was the leadership of the

IOM and the people who worked on the report, entitled *To Err Is Human: Building a Safer Health System,* that gave the American public the first glimpse of the underbelly of America's health system.

This is good news because, in many hospitals, when a patient dies from a medical mistake, the mistake is either covered up or ignored, and it's back to business as usual. A review of the events might occur, a few staff might be reprimanded, an underling might be fired. As one nurse said, "If they could get away with it, they would try to cover it up."

Rarely do hospitals or other health care facilities look to find the root causes of medical mistakes and change the policies and practices that cause them. And even more rare are health care organizations that proactively look for mistakes waiting to happen and correct those practices that can lead to mistakes—even by the most conscientious and careful doctor, nurse, or pharmacist. Most health care executives, physicians, and hospital board members don't know the number of deaths and serious injuries that occur in their own facilities as a result of preventable medical mistakes.

This begs an even bigger question: How many of them ask? If they don't seek, they won't find. If they don't find, they can't fix what's wrong.

Big Business Tallies the Toll of Mistakes

When word of the IOM report hit the public airwaves, officials at General Motors estimated how many of its 1.25 million employees, retirees, and their family members might be affected by medical mistakes. Using the national estimates as a basis, GM calculated that about 488 of its employees, retirees, and family members die every year from medical mistakes. Bruce Bradley of General Motors said, "Every day, we could be losing between one and two employees as a result of medical error."[5] Imagine what would happen if that many GM employees died each week from on-the-job accidents.

Today, when a GM employee dies or is severely injured while on the job, the company shuts down operations at the plant where the accident occurred until investigators can determine what went wrong. In fact, that's the rule of thumb among most American companies. When a fatal or life-threatening accident occurs, business as usual comes to a halt, the cause of the accident is determined, and actions are taken to prevent it from happening again. Now GM and other big businesses across the nation are taking action to prevent their employees and retirees from bearing the consequences of mistakes and poor-quality health care, and exerting pressure on health care organizations to make mistakes as rare as possible.

Cracks in the Wall

Many doctors and nurses privately express deep concern about medical mistakes, yet they remain silent. If they speak out publicly, their jobs and professional standing may be at risk.

Many, if not all, have a story to tell about medical mistakes or near misses they were involved in or witnessed. And for conscientious health care professionals, the harm caused is often devastating. The memory of those mistakes haunts them for the remainder of their careers. Some quietly leave to earn a living doing something else.

Ilene says that Michael's surgeon was probably heartsick about what happened to her son. But she'll never really know how he felt because the wall of silence between doctor and patient precludes honest and open communication about such a tragedy.

Even physicians and nurses who are leaders in their fields and have spent their careers trying to improve the quality of health care are unable to make the system work safely and effectively for themselves, their spouses, their parents, and their children. Thus, the story of medical mistakes is not an "us" and "them" story. We're all in the same boat.

In fact, one physician leader, Dr. Mark Chassin, has asked the public for its help. In an article in the *Journal of the American Medical Association,* he writes that Americans need to "press to keep quality care at the top of the agenda and to seek effective ways for health care professionals, administrators and others to be accountable to patients and society for the quality of care."[6]

So Much Good, but Not Good Enough

The health care system does so much good for so many people when they are sick and injured. Certainly, it's not the case that the next visit to your doctor has to be scary or dangerous. In fact, many of the people who have stories to tell about medical mistakes also have glowing praise for those doctors and nurses who *are* competent and compassionate, honest, and open, and who helped repair the damage caused by medical mistakes.

Dedicated physicians, nurses, and researchers have worked diligently to improve the safety of many common medical procedures. Heart surgery, for example, has become much safer, and mortality rates continue to decline. This reduction in mortality has occurred because of scrupulous attention to surgical technique and practice, as well as advances in technology.

Over the past fifteen years, the number of anesthesia-related deaths has fallen dramatically. Some of this improvement is due to better drugs and devices to monitor the effects of anesthesia on a patient. But much of the improvement came about because anesthesiologists took time to study the root causes of deaths and make changes in the basic setup of the operating room that make it impossible for some of the most critical mistakes to occur at all.

These improvements reflect the underlying ethic of medicine in its most profound and satisfying form, and they symbolize why the American health care system is the world's envy. Television news regularly broadcasts stories of new treatments and new discoveries about diseases and their causes. Americans are hungry for anything that sparks hope for a cure for the multitude of diseases that disable and kill us. We are accustomed to advances in medicine and the miracles they bring. Our expectation for new discovery is born from the hope and optimism that is uniquely American. We expect advances that allow the blind to see, the dying to live. Now, surgeons operate on fetuses in the womb to fuse the spine and prevent a child from living a life with crippling spina bifida. Americans don't ask *if* there will be a cure for Alzheimer's disease. Instead, we ask *when*.

But what good are new discoveries and cures learned from the great work of scientists if they are misapplied and patients die or are injured while being treated with wonder medicine? With what kind of reverence are we treating this human body? Walt Whitman once said, "If anything is sacred the human body is sacred." Are we doing justice to this vessel?

There are no guarantees when it comes to health care. Every human body is different, and a treatment that is successful for one person may be unsuccessful for another. Some people might have a bad reaction to a newly prescribed drug that is appropriately prescribed. The bad reaction is unknowable in advance and isn't the result of a medical mistake. Rather, it is evidence of how much remains unknown about the human body and how to treat diseases that afflict it. We can only hope that medical knowledge will continue to progress and that others, in the future, will not suffer the same fate.

But when a physician prescribes a medication for a patient whose allergy to that drug is known and documented, *that* is a preventable medical mistake. Similarly, when it is known that bleeding after a tonsillectomy is a warning sign, and when those warning signs are repeatedly ignored, *that* is a preventable medical mistake.

What the health care system gives with one hand, it must not take away with the other. It is not enough to improve surgical procedures or enhance medical knowledge. Even weeding out incompetent health care professionals won't solve the problem. Making health care safer requires changing how health care is organized and how health professionals work together and communicate. Though actions by individual doctors, nurses, and pharmacists are often the apparent cause of medical mistakes, many are the result of a culmination of errors. They result from a problem in the "system" of care, the chain of literally hundreds of actions by doctors, nurses, technicians, pharmacists, and others who are involved in the care of a patient. This is the Achilles' heel of modern medicine, where so many professionals care for the same patient, yet communication among them is poor. In Michael's case, the warning signs were never communicated to the surgeon on the day he couldn't be reached. And he probably never got word of Ilene's sweatshirt caked with blood.

2 | The Human Face
of Medical Mistakes

People from all walks of life are affected by medical mistakes: Gulf War veterans, doctors, store managers, nurses, real estate agents, automobile assembly line workers, high school athletes, first-graders. Each has a story to tell that is profoundly moving. These stories are not easy to hear, but they are a window into how the medical system fails us and the enormity of the impact. Human stories touch the heart and the mind and translate national statistics into the reality of day-to-day life.

From time to time, newspaper accounts have conveyed stories that relay the key facts about medical mistakes, as in the case of a six-year-old boy who died at a New York hospital while undergoing a magnetic resonance imaging (MRI) test. Somehow, a metal oxygen canister about the size of a fire extinguisher was mistakenly brought into the room where the test was under way. The MRI machine contains a powerful magnet that pulls any metal object toward it with tremendous force. According to an account by the *New York Times*, the oxygen tank flew to the magnet at a speed of twenty to thirty feet per second. The little boy's skull was fractured and he died. The hospital was fined $22,000, the maximum allowed by law.

What lies beneath the cold, hard facts? What happens to the families, to the survivors? Beneath the facts are the other sides to the stories. There's the heartbreak and loneliness of husbands and wives who have spent a lifetime together, only to have one of them left behind to mourn the loss of their lifelong companion. There are the husbands and wives who divorce because the grief over the injury their child sustained is too great. The guilt—that somehow the medical mistake was their fault, that they didn't do the one thing that could have prevented what had happened to their child—is beyond repair.

For others, disfiguring physical scars from multiple surgeries to repair mistakes cause them to lie awake in the middle of the night wondering whether they will ever find a mate who will love them for who they are inside, not for what is on the outside. And others tell stories of stellar careers they spent years building, only to see them come to a crashing halt because they could no longer work. All of these are stories of people who have lost a part of themselves. That part may be a loved one, or a physical part of their body, or their identity and sense of self.

A Cry to Be Heard

Why tell the stories behind medical mistakes? Many people who have borne the consequences of preventable medical mistakes want their stories told. In fact, the sad part of writing this book is that there were too many stories to tell, too many people who wanted to share the depth of their pain and let the world know how bad the health care system can be.

For some, the desire to tell their story is part of the healing process. A thirty-five-year-old mother of two boys who is living with horrible consequences of a botched elective procedure said, "Every time I tell my story, I feel better. I am educating somebody by telling others. I am giving them fair warning." For others, telling their stories to sympathetic listeners validates what they have seen, heard, and done.

Unlike airplane crashes, medical mistakes happen quietly, one at a time. They are tragedies that occur unnoticed. The federal government counts the number of people who die in plane crashes, who die from drunk driving accidents, and who die from diseases like cancer and AIDS. But no one counts the number of people who die from medical mistakes. No national mourning or outpouring of sympathy occurs, making it seem as if the profound effects of mistakes don't matter and no one cares. Powerful forces in the health care industry want to keep this silence unbroken.

Even when those who have experienced errors try to tell their stories, willing listeners may be hard to find. Some people don't want to hear about medical mistakes or don't believe they can happen. One person says, "People put a lot of wishful thinking into their doctor and the system, and they don't want to hear about what can go wrong."

A nurse whose mother died after she was given an overdose of a medication says how important it is for people to tell their stories. She advises others who have been through experiences similar to hers to, "Tell people, talk about it. Some may not understand it, but others will. The validation is so important. It's like gold."

Another daughter wrote to say that she tells the story of her father's death from a medical mistake because she wants the American public to know that medical mistakes are an "epidemic that faces our nation." She goes on to say, "We are the voices of the thousands of individuals who have lost their lives to medical mistakes." Yet another daughter says, "I love to tell my story as much as possible. It makes me feel as if my father had a purpose in dying."

Finally, by telling these stories, we hope that others will come forward and tell theirs. As Mary, an Emmy Award-winning television anchor and victim of a horrible mistake, says, "There will be so many coming forward that they will blacken the sky and you won't see the sun. I say this not as a patient, but as a journalist who has covered health care."

■ **OCKIE, WORLD WAR II VETERAN**

A World War II Army veteran and part of the greatest generation that served our country, Ockie relished life. He was a retired golf pro who worked seven days a week at a local golf club. His daughter says, "He was the kind of man you were proud to say was your father. He loved us and provided for us."

A strong, energetic seventy-five-year-old husband and father of four, Ockie never needed more than five hours of sleep a night. He was diagnosed with esophageal cancer after coughing up blood one morning before his daily golf outing. In otherwise excellent health, he was prepared to undergo the necessary chemotherapy and radiation therapy as a prelude to having surgery to remove what ended up being a small residual tumor. Ockie weathered the brutal therapy, rebuilt his strength, and was in good shape for the complicated surgery, which he sailed through on a Friday in October 1998. The surgeon remarked afterward how pleased he was with the operation and how well his patient had tolerated the six-and-a-half-hour procedure.

Over the next three days, Ockie was making a strong recovery from the surgery. He remained in the intensive care unit during this time because the surgeon had inserted a nasogastric (NG) tube, which goes through a patient's nose and into his stomach. It removes any gastric secretions in the days after the surgery.

On the morning of the fourth day after surgery, Ockie's daughter, Rebecca, drove her mother, Geri, to the hospital, just as she had done the previous three days. It was approximately 10:15 A.M. when the two women turned a corner to enter his room and saw a crowd of doctors and nurses assembled around Ockie's bed. One of them escorted mother and daughter to a nearby waiting room. While the two waited and were thinking the worst, the hospital chaplain arrived, and shortly afterward, so did Ockie's surgeon, who was angry and devastated. He told Rebecca and Geri that Ockie's NG tube had somehow come out. He threw his hands up in the air and stormed out of the room.

The family only later realized the significance of what had happened. During the surgery, the NG tube was placed through Ockie's nose and extended to the tip of his stomach. After the NG tube had somehow come out, a nurse had reinserted it—incorrectly—through his vocal cords and into his lungs, *despite the doctor's written orders that the tube should not be repositioned if it did come out.* Ockie developed bacterial pneumonia and was now in critical condition.

When Rebecca and her mom finally got to see Ockie, they were aghast: he had looked so good the night before, and now he appeared comatose, hooked up to life support. It was immediately clear that an anticipated ten- to fourteen-day hospital stay was going to stretch on far longer. Little did they know that Ockie would never go home. He lingered in the intensive care unit for over four months, receiving massive amounts of potent antibiotics in an attempt to stem the infection that was ravaging his body.

Throughout most of the ordeal, Ockie was alert and knew something was terribly wrong. He kept mouthing the words, "What the hell happened?" His wife and family were too afraid to tell him the truth, fearing that if he knew, he wouldn't let another doctor or nurse come near him. "After a while, he didn't look like our father any more," Rebecca says. The sparkle that was always in his eyes was gone.

Ockie died in March 1999, one hundred and thirty-nine days after entering the hospital. His kidneys finally failed as a result of the powerful drugs he had been given to fight the bacterial pneumonia. Just three months shy of his fiftieth wedding anniversary, Ockie was buried. His daughter says, "He didn't deserve to die the way he did. He deserved to die when his time was due. My dad should have died in his sleep or from fighting a disease, not from a mistake."

Geri, Ockie's wife and soul mate, is lonely, devastated, and angry. She now lives alone in a small cottage just behind her daughter's house. To this day she wonders how it could be that the hospital has never offered her an apology and would not step up to the plate and help after they made the mistake that led to the death of her husband of almost fifty years. She wrote to us and said, "I hope and pray this never has to happen to another family. We need hospitals to speak up and tell the family a mistake was made and consult with them to explain what happened. This would have meant a great deal to me and would have helped in the healing process."

■ **DANIEL, WHITE HOUSE OFFICIAL**

Daniel is a brilliant man who devoted his life to public service. A graduate of one of the country's elite universities and the nation's leading business school, he was in his twenties when he started working in the White House. He earned two Presidential letters of commendation, and was twenty-nine years old when he earned the Distinguished Civilian Service Award. He worked fourteen-hour days in the Old Executive Office Building, commuting from his home in a Washington, D.C., suburb.

The picture of health, Daniel was thirty-four years old when he had elective surgery on his jaw, which he later found out wasn't even necessary. The outcome of the surgery was disastrous, and he suffered profound damage to his cranial nerves as a result of mistakes made by the surgeon. His life came to a screeching halt—a brilliant career destroyed. He is disabled and suffers excruciating pain in the regions from his ears to his chin and eyes. Irritable bowel syndrome, which he didn't have before the surgery, prevents him from going to the bathroom normally. Diabetes accompanied the irritable bowel syndrome; his vision, too, is impaired.

"I've lost six teeth and the rest are severely damaged," he told us. He goes on to say, "I dwell in anguish. If you ask me what my pain is on the pain scale, it's off the charts virtually all the time. It is almost impossible for me to do any work. If I have an hour a day that is good, it is a good day. I would rather live with this than to have caused this to anyone." Daniel reflects on how medical mistakes can devastate families. "It has prevented me from getting married to my fiancée and starting a family."

Daniel's story stops here because he can't say any more. After nine years, he is still making a brave effort to hold the system accountable for what happened to him. The cost of treatment for all the ailments caused by one botched procedure has totaled hundreds of thousands of dollars. He says, "Insurance covered some of it, but you are lucky to get fifty-five cents on the dollar. And then there's lost income and travel costs to doctors' offices. When doctors ask me what I do for a living," Daniel quips, "I say I am a Mercedes salesman. They ask about the location of the dealership and I say, 'Well, I just put cars in doctors' driveways.' It's true. My medical expenses have paid for many, though I am lucky when I can drive at all." More sobering, though, he says, "If I didn't have resources to cope, I don't see how I could have survived to this point."

■ **MARY, EMMY AWARD-WINNING TELEVISION NEWS ANCHOR**

A seven-time Emmy Award winner, Chicago-based television news anchor, and journalist, Mary traveled the world. She reported from Poland on the Solidarity Movement as it was taking hold and the Communist regime was falling. Later, as head of her own communications company, she was a leading force in creating one of the nation's most successful health campaigns, Breast Cancer Awareness Month. Despite her awards and accomplishments, a cold fact of the television news business is that youth sells, and at age forty-two, Mary decided to have cosmetic surgery to help her remain at the top of her profession. Unfortunately, that was a decision that stopped her career dead in its tracks.

As soon as she awoke from a seven-and-a-half-hour outpatient procedure, performed by a reputable physician, she knew something disastrous had happened. "I didn't think it was possible to have that much pain and be conscious," she says. Later, Mary recalls that one of her other doctors told her father, "Imagine you have all of your fingers and toes amputated without anesthesia. Now imagine having that pain every day. This is the amount of pain Mary has." This is the physical pain she has endured for more than eight years.

To this day, Mary and her current doctors don't know what went wrong. "There were four people in the room," she says, "the doctor, the nurse, the anesthesiologist, and me. Two of them worked for the doctor and they wouldn't say anything about what went wrong."

The cosmetic procedure ended Mary's illustrious career. Her husband left her. To pay her medical bills, she had to sell her house and her engagement ring. The fine print of her insurance policy stated that it would not cover the cost of two things: injuries incurred during the commission of a felony and pain from cosmetic procedures. The initial cost of pain treatment for six months was $65,000. Today she pays $2,000 a month just for prescriptions for her pain medication, and this will probably go on for the rest of her life. Mary says, "I don't want an apology from the doctor, but I do want him to dismiss the huge medical bills."

Her life changed forever, Mary can no longer do the simple things others take for granted. She can't go visit a friend or go to the ballet. "Today," she says, "I couldn't walk out my front door. But at least I could get to the kitchen. Yesterday, I couldn't get out of bed."

■ ELIZABETH, AN EIGHT-YEAR-OLD WISE BEYOND HER YEARS

When eight-year-old Elizabeth told her parents that her kidney cancer, which had been in remission, was back, her parents believed her. She was experiencing severe pain in her legs that only morphine could relieve. But the little girl's doctors dismissed her complaints as psychological, stemming from her fear of the cancer recurring. Though Elizabeth had been scheduled for an MRI, the test was canceled because the doctors thought it wasn't necessary. As her mother, Leila, recalled, "The doctors said that my daughter was being manipulative and that I was only raising her anxiety by continuing to take her to doctors." Leila did everything she could not to reinforce Elizabeth's complaints about pain, believing the doctors' view that all was well and that her daughter's cancer phobia needed to be overcome, not encouraged. Leila recalls with a profound sadness how she insisted one Christmas morning that her daughter crawl down the stairs to open presents despite her cries for relief from her pain.

Over the next three months, Elizabeth's symptoms worsened and she lost almost twenty pounds, going from fifty-eight to forty pounds. Her mom called the doctors about twenty more times, and they continued to assure her that her daughter's troubles were in her head. Elizabeth continued to worsen and became totally withdrawn, not talking to anyone; her doctor had her placed in an outpatient psychiatric ward. Meanwhile, "She just laid there with her eyes closed," her mom says.

With the instinct that only a parent has, Leila called her own mother and said, "Her soul is dying. There is no life in her eyes." She was right. No one knew—not yet—that Elizabeth's brain was swelling because a tumor had metastasized to her spine and was in her brain, pressing on it. On the morning of the day she was finally diagnosed, her dad asked her what she was thinking about, and she replied, "I'm thinking about heaven. There's no pain there."

Later that day she had a seizure. Her doctors ordered an MRI, which proved what Elizabeth had known in her heart all along. The cancer had spread to her spine and brain. Nine months of chemotherapy and a stem cell transplant saved Elizabeth's life, but the delay in diagnosis resulted in permanent paralysis from the waist down.

The little girl, a wise and sensitive child, wanted to ask her doctors why they did not believe her when she said her cancer had come back. None would agree to meet with her and talk to her, and only one of the five ever apologized. One day when her parents were distraught, she said to her mother, with the wisdom that a child holds, "I forgive you, Mom, but you have to forgive yourself."

■ SUSAN, FINANCIAL MANAGER

Susan underwent a laparoscopic procedure to check for an ovarian cyst and ended up having four additional surgeries to repair the damage done in the first procedure. One of the risks of this procedure is that the surgeon can accidentally puncture a major organ. Susan's surgeon did inform her of this possibility; however, the surgeon played down the risk and gave Susan what she says was a false sense of confidence.

After the procedure, Susan says, "I was discharged home the same day and was sick to my stomach. I thought it was the anesthesia. That night I couldn't sleep and the next morning I had a lot of abdominal pain." Two of Susan's friends were taking care of her and they started calling the doctor at 8 o'clock the next morning. The doctor returned the call around noon and said the pain was a normal reaction after the procedure and that Susan should have some lunch and take some of the pain medication she had been prescribed. "By 3 P.M. I was dripping with sweat and the pain was an eleven on a scale of one to ten," she recalls. "My friends were ready to call nine-one-one, but instead, there I was, in my nightgown and robe and slippers, and my two friends helping me get in the car."

They rushed her to the emergency department. After seven hours of tests and waiting for results, the doctor on duty realized Susan was in serious trouble and ordered emergency surgery. During the laparoscopic procedure, the doctor had punctured Susan's colon, and she developed peritonitis, a severe and life-threatening infection of the central body cavity that develops when the intestines or colon are punctured, leaking their bacteria-loaded contents into the body cavity. The emergency surgeon could not repair the colon, so he flushed out her body cavity, removed the damaged part of the colon, and performed a temporary colostomy, in which the colon is connected to a waste-collection bag through a hole created in the abdomen.

When Susan awoke after surgery, she was incredibly angry. "To wake and find you have a bag attached to your body collecting feces…the nurses kept coming to try to teach me how to empty it, and I just refused," she said. "I was so bitter about the colostomy." Susan remained in the hospital for a month and eventually required more surgeries to correct all the problems caused by the initial mistake. She lost five months of work, and her medical bills surpassed $150,000, $15,000 of which she had to cover herself. She didn't have the money to pay the bills, so she charged them on her credit cards. Fortunately for Susan, she worked for a large company that had generous medical and disability benefits, and that stood by her throughout the ordeal. "If I had worked for a small business, there's no way they could have kept me on," she says with an obvious sense of relief.

But the effects of this mistake are more profound than time lost and debt incurred. Susan recently found out that she will have discomfort and problems going to the bathroom for the rest of her life. More personally, Susan, a single woman, now has terrible scars on her abdomen. "It's horrid, a daily reminder," she says. "There's a fear of intimacy now. I don't want to get undressed in front of someone."

■ MARION, MOTHER AND REAL ESTATE AGENT

Marion was an energetic, optimistic, bright and cheery woman who, three months before she died from a medication overdose while in the hospital, was on a cruise, dancing and having the time of her life. Her daughter, Patti, is a nurse practitioner who prides herself on providing excellent care to her patients. With amazement, she says,

"I can't tell you how many times I have seen careless errors and watched them be covered up without a morsel of conscience." Little did she know that her mother would succumb to a preventable medical mistake.

It was on a hot July 4th, not long after Marion returned home from vacation, that she started complaining of unrelenting gas and abdominal pain after eating. Patti was worried about this unusual and sudden change and drove her mom to the hospital emergency department. The ER doctor told Patti that all the tests results were normal and that her mom was just having a gall bladder attack. Patti told the doctor that her mother's gall bladder had been removed years earlier, and she asked if other tests could be performed before her mother was discharged. The doctor abruptly left the bedside, walked down the hall, and minutes later, motioned Patti to follow. Patti recalls the doctor saying, "I had forgotten to look at the X-rays we did until you just asked me about them." A white spot was found in Marion's lung. The doctor admitted her to the hospital for evaluation, which revealed a cancerous mass that had spread to her liver.

Marion asked, "All I want to know is whether or not there is any chance that I can beat this." The surgeon said that surgery was not a good option, but she could try chemotherapy. Patti then said, "You need to know that my mother is a very optimistic and determined person who has a history of beating the odds." The surgeon said he had seen more aggressive cancers, and those patients had survived and beaten the odds. As Patti recalls, her mom replied, "That's all I need to know."

While at home awaiting her scheduled appointment for a second opinion at a local cancer hospital to discuss treatment options, Marion was still unable to eat or drink anything without another long bout of belching. Patti drove her mom back to the local hospital and she was admitted; later, she was transferred to the cancer hospital where she would soon have her outpatient appointment.

While Marion was in the hospital the next day, the nurse came and gave her medication for her belching and her pain, which made her sleep for hours. Worried about how groggy and confused her mom was, Patti asked the doctor if her mom could have medication that wouldn't make her so sleepy. But despite Patti's protestations, the doctor increased the dose of pain medication that was making her mom groggy. Later, Patti went back to her mother's room and tried to wake her up, and she did wake up, albeit slowly. Worried about the reaction her mom had to the current drug regimen, she asked the doctor—and he agreed—to let Marion stay one more night and be discharged the following morning in time for her outpatient appointment.

This was the fateful day, the one extra day in the hospital that Patti will never forget. After arriving at the hospital that night, Patti found her mom asleep. At 2 A.M., the nurse tried to wake Marion. Patti went to her mother's bedside, repeating over and over, "Ma, wake up, it's me, Patti," to no avail. Marion lay motionless, like dead weight. Patti asked the nurse to get the doctor, but got no response. She couldn't fathom how the doctor and nurse could say everything is okay when her mom couldn't wake up. (Patti later found out that this incident was not reported in her mother's medical record.)

Patti recalls, "I was desperate over what I should do. I debated calling nine-one-one—from my mother's room—just to get her out of there and into the hands of someone who knew what they were doing." Her experience told her that her mother was showing the signs of respiratory depression. She questioned the medications and doses but, as she said, they just "blew me off." A half-hour later, the nurse returned and told Patti that the doctor said "for you to just not be so anxious."

Patti says her mother was given too much morphine for pain—despite the fact that her mother had no complaints about significant pain from her newly diagnosed cancer. Her mom was given medication to reverse the effects of the morphine, and Patti describes what she saw next. Her mom woke up, and through waves of tears, Patti recalls, "All I could do was watch her die. Sitting straight up in bed, her baby blue eyes had no pupils and she didn't recognize me. She kept screaming over and over in a baby-like voice, 'Momma, Daddy, help me,' like a two-year-old girl."

Looking back on these horrifying events, Patti says, "I should have let her go home but I was afraid to bring her home. I made them keep her an extra day. I live with the memories of this nightmare almost every minute of every day and will for the rest of my life. They just wouldn't listen. I will never forgive myself for not protecting my mother from this horrible fate; my greatest mistake was that I did not stop them. I stayed alive only because my mother, and father for that matter, wouldn't have liked it if I had quit."

◼ DIANA, FORMER AIR FORCE INTELLIGENCE OFFICER

As an Air Force intelligence officer, Diana was physically fit and kept in good shape, working out regularly despite chronic hip pain that eventually drove her to see her doctor. He diagnosed her as having severe osteoarthritis and recommended a total hip replacement to correct the damage. Only thirty-nine years old at the time, she debated whether to have the procedure. She decided to go ahead with the surgery and scheduled it with a physician who was a partner in a prestigious orthopedic hospital. The surgery went well. But the week that Diana was admitted, her surgeon's partners, along with their trained orthopedic staff, transferred their practice to another hospital. Diana's surgeon remained and became chief of staff of the hospital's skeletal and unmotivated crew.

After the surgery, Diana awoke to find a tray of cold food on a chair across the room and no sign of nursing staff. She pushed the nurse's button—she was in excruciating pain and had been without pain relief for hours—but no nurse arrived. The next day, her break-fast, lunch, and dinner trays were delivered and again left on a chair across the room, where she could not reach them. The button to the nurse's station still had not been connected, and she could not call anyone to help her get her meals. Outraged by the substandard care, Diana's friends demanded that she be transferred to the hospital where the surgeon's partners had relocated. She was transferred to the new hospital the next day and expected to be put under the care of her surgeon's partners and their trained orthopedic staff. Instead, her surgeon insisted that an osteopathic physician, whose specialty was brain and spinal injuries, oversee her care.

Her first night in the new hospital was not much better. She buzzed the nursing staff for help walking to the bathroom. It seemed that no nurses were on duty that evening in the head trauma unit where she was assigned, but a male medical techni-cian responded. Weak from the surgery and dizzy, she fainted. The medical technician managed to catch her before she hit the floor, and he helped her back into bed, though he made only a cursory notation about the incident in her chart, since the standard proce-dure in that ward was to report only those falls that involved a patient's head actually hitting the floor.

By the next evening, Diana's hip was so painful that she couldn't sit up without crying out in pain. She recalls, "The spasms were so severe in my leg and hip joint that it felt as if my leg was being torn out of my body." Her surgeon was out of town, and the osteopathic physician dismissed her pain as "hypersensitivity" and prescribed more frequent doses of painkillers. Though she wouldn't learn this for another six weeks, when she had her first postoperative exam with the surgeon, she had actually dislocated the new joint when she fell and was lifted back into the bed by the medical technician.

On the day she was discharged from the hospital, Diana was instructed to take a taxi to her surgeon's office for her first checkup; she hadn't seen him since the day of surgery. The surgeon took an X-ray, which revealed that the ball of the implant had buried itself several inches out of place, and scar tissue had formed around the ball, creating a "false socket." Two more surgeries that week to get the implant back into the socket and Diana was back where she had started six weeks earlier, but in a greatly weakened state. "Were I not young, fit, and healthy, I believe I would have died," she said later.

But luck evidently wasn't with Diana, for during her second stint at rehabilitation in the same hospital, the physical therapist dropped her leg off the side of her wheelchair while he tried to reattach her leg brace. This time, however, Diana was going to speak up for herself. The same osteopathic physician who had belittled her pain earlier refused to take an X-ray, but Diana adamantly demanded it. Sure enough, her new hip had been dislocated *again*, requiring a fourth surgery. To prevent further mishaps, the orthopedic surgeon enclosed her in a full body cast and shipped her off to a nursing home for another six weeks. Once again, the surgeon never came to see her during this time.

Her travails were still not over. Two weeks after starting rehabilitation for a third time, she began to lose the ability to move her leg, and her hip started throbbing with a dull, aching pain. The orthopedic surgeon dismissed her as a complainer and would not discuss her condition with her. At this point, Diana decided to seek a second opinion, this time from the senior orthopedic surgeon at a prestigious university medical center. The X-rays he took did not bear good news. The muscle and other soft tissue around the new hip joint had been so badly damaged that there was nothing he could do for two years, and even then, there was a chance she would never walk without a steel brace or crutches.

In June 1995, nearly two years after what was supposed to be a routine hip replacement, Diana had the needed surgery at a hospital with a track record of working to improve the safety of patient care, and this time there were no complications afterward. Seven years later, in July 2002, Diana had another surgery because the hip implant was wearing out. But because the surgery and follow-up care were so good, she says, "In just ten weeks, I started swimming again, and biking, walking, weight training, and yoga. I'm so grateful that I found my voice to speak up for myself."

■ LEWIS, FIFTEEN-YEAR-OLD STUDENT, TOP IN HIS CLASS

By all accounts, Lewis was a child who any parent would be so proud to call their son. A top student, he ranked in the highest 1 percent of his age group nationwide. He was a prize-winning mathematical contestant, a budding writer who reported for the youth section of his local newspaper, and an experienced actor who regularly appeared in community stage and television productions. He already had a touch of national fame, having appeared in a television commercial at age seven with the late NASCAR legend, Dale Earnhardt.

Lewis was born with his breastbone sunken into the chest cavity, a condition called pectus excavatum. The condition affects as many as one in five hundred children, and some doctors believe that it may interfere with the ability of the lungs to expand fully and, if not corrected, might lead to respiratory problems later on. Lewis's parents saw an article in their local paper that described in glowing terms a new surgical procedure to correct the defect. In this procedure a metal bar is inserted through three small incisions in the chest, and the bar props up the breastbone. The article described the surgery as an advance over surgery that requires opening the whole chest cavity and indicated that most patients have a quick, easy recovery.

Lewis and his parents spoke to a surgeon at a hospital affiliated with the state's prestigious medical school about the surgery. Having confidence in the reputation of both hospital and surgeon, they decided to go ahead with the procedure. His mom, Helen, noted in the journal she wrote after Lewis's death, "We thought it was like getting braces."

The surgery was on a Thursday and took much longer than Lewis's parents had anticipated, but the surgeon assured them that Lewis had done well throughout. After the surgery Lewis was given pain medication through an epidural line in his back. In addition, he was given regular injections of a powerful painkiller that was labeled with warnings in bold print about the possibility of perforated ulcers, bleeding, and kidney failure—a sign that any patient taking the medication should be closely monitored.

From the recovery room, Lewis was moved to the children's cancer ward because no beds were available in the pediatric surgery ward. Lewis's doctor had the weekend off, but another surgeon checked on Lewis on Saturday morning, two days after surgery. This was the last seasoned physician who would see Lewis until his death two days later. He noted no evidence of infection and said that Lewis was doing well enough to get out of bed.

Early Sunday morning, Lewis was suddenly stricken by over-whelming pain in his stomach, the "worst pain imaginable," he told his mom. Helen called in a nurse, who told her that it was just gas pain, and even though the boy claimed his pain was five on a scale of five, the nurse said he just needed to get up and walk around. Later, another nurse suggested a bath. At the nurse's insis-tence, Lewis, supported on either side by his mom and the nurse, took a very painful walk around the floor, with Lewis stopping every few steps. Only later would Lewis's family know that the pain was the first warning sign of a perforated duodenal ulcer, a known and stated risk of the powerful medication he was given. The ulcer was eating a hole in his upper intestine, allowing toxic fluids to flow into his abdominal cavity.

By Sunday afternoon, Lewis was beginning to show signs of incipient shock, a life-threatening medical emergency caused by blood loss and infection. The boy's belly was bloated, his pulse was rising, his temperature had dropped, and he was pale and weak, dripping with cold sweat. The nurse continued to insist that Lewis was not walking enough to rid himself of gas pain, and they took another agonizing walk, and another bath. But for most of the afternoon, Helen said, "I hunched over the bed with Lewis gripping my hand in pain."

Helen repeatedly asked the nurses to call a doctor to examine her son. Each time, instead of a full-fledged doctor, an exhausted-looking first-year resident arrived. Finally, Helen demanded that the nurse call either the original surgeon, the doctor who examined Lewis on Saturday morning, or one of their partners on call. The nurse was exasperated and the resident clearly offended. Helen wrote in her journal, "She is offended, and appears extremely downcast that I have questioned her judgment. I feel bad for her. To stand my ground, I reiterate Lewis's alarming symptoms once again. She stands at the computer and nods glumly, but never says a word. My impression is that she is too angry to speak."

Apparently, no seasoned doctor was ever called. On Sunday evening, hours after Helen's request, another young doctor arrived. Helen assumed this is the veteran doctor she had requested. In fact, he is another resident. A fourth-year resident, he has more training and experience than the neophyte first-year resident, but is still under the supervision of a seasoned physician.

Again, Lewis's mom was told that the excruciating abdominal pain is from constipation due to the pain medications. The resident recorded a heart rate of 80 beats per minute, but a nurse who took the boy's pulse ten minutes earlier had recorded it as an elevated 126 beats per minute. The results of a blood test that came back about midnight showed the first signs of a deadly imbalance that can shut down the body's vital organs. Lewis's mom noted, "No one put these clues together." The critical blood tests, those that would check for infection and blood loss, were not performed.

That night, Lewis's heart rate soared to 142 beats per minute. His temperature dropped to 95 degrees. Helen wrote in her journal, "Neither Lewis nor I sleep at all Sunday night. I have given up on the weekend staff and am waiting for the morning when the regular staff and doctors arrive. But their arrival simply brings confusion. Nothing is coordinated, no one seems to be in charge of the care."

Despite his alarming symptoms, Lewis had received no special monitoring through the night. Then, on Monday morning, an aide taking routine vital signs was unable to get a blood pressure reading. For about two hours, nurses tried to take Lewis's blood pressure and could not get a reading. They tried repeatedly with an assortment of blood pressure cuffs, believing they couldn't get a reading because the devices were broken. His mom says, "No one seemed concerned that this might be an emergency requiring immediate action." Finally, on the seventh blood pressure cuff, a second-year resident thought she detected a reading of 110/58. The staff, satisfied, now had something to write down in the boy's chart. A sign of massive internal bleeding, stemming from the perforated ulcer, was missed.

That morning, Lewis's pain in his abdomen suddenly stops. The nurses think this is a positive sign. In fact, in a situation such as this, sudden cessation of abdominal pain can be a sign of imminent death. Meanwhile, Lewis catches a glimpse of himself in the mirror and says, "My God. I am the same color as the sheets," Helen wrote.

Later that fateful Monday morning, Lewis told his mom that the world was going black. It's the last thing he ever said. "Ish... going...black." It's going black. He repeats it again and passes out. His mom wrote, "Suddenly Lewis is dead. It is 12:05 P.M. His father and little sister are watching in horror from the back of the room. I run out of the room crying for help. I have never seen someone die before, much less my own, perfectly healthy child."

The fourth-year resident appeared again, and when he couldn't revive the boy, he called a "code," a full alert that a patient is in imminent danger of dying. Residents and—finally—seasoned physicians streamed into the room. But of course by then it was too late. After trying to revive Lewis for an hour and a half, the doctors pronounced him dead, thirty-one hours after his symptoms began.

When Lewis's parents called family members to tell them what had happened, they described his symptoms over the past twenty-four hours. Helen wrote, "My cousin, an internist, suspects a perforated ulcer or sepsis. My brother, an attorney, looks up the symptoms in the Mayo Handbook [from the prestigious Mayo Medical Clinic in Rochester, Minnesota] and he independently reaches the same conclusion." The autopsy results reported the same diagnosis. Three liters of blood and other fluids were found in Lewis's abdomen. A boy of Lewis's age has only four to five liters of blood.

A subsequent review of Lewis's case concluded that there had been many clear indications of the gravity of Lewis's condition, and that the nurses and residents should have summoned an experienced doctor at any one of many points throughout the boy's ordeal. If they had done so, a simple blood test would have shown the infection and internal bleeding that led to his death. An experienced physician who reviewed Lewis's medical record was quoted in a local newspaper, *The State*, on June 16, 2002, as saying, "Even a Boy Scout could have done better. It's hard to kill a healthy 15-year-old."

■ MADELINE, GRANDMOTHER WITH THE WILL TO LIVE

Seventy-five-year-old Madeline fractured her hip in a fall at home, but even her daughter Donna's credentials as a nurse couldn't save Madeline from a medical mistake that has left her unable to walk without pain. Madeline had surgery to repair the fracture—a relatively common procedure in older people—and was sent home with a walker after a month in the hospital.

Although her orthopedic surgeon assured her that she was healing properly, Madeline continued to have severe pain from her hip to her foot. In fact, she was unable to place her foot flat on the floor without experiencing sharp pain in her repaired hip. After three days of this, Madeline went back to the emergency department, where her hip was X-rayed and her surgeon once again assured her that her hip was healing well.

Six days later, Madeline was admitted to a rehabilitation center. Since the surgery, she had lost twenty-five pounds off an already slight frame—20 percent of her body weight—and was unable to get out of bed because of the pain. She had also developed blood clots in her leg.

Concerned about her mother's lack of progress, Donna traveled to Florida to visit her in the rehabilitation center. She recalls, "My mother was extremely depressed and crying. I slept alongside my mother in the bed that night, but we didn't really sleep. She kept saying, 'There is something poking me, it's like a knife. Look in the bed, there's something there.' I looked and there was nothing there. I was so desperate and tried so hard not to cry." Very early the next morning, Donna called an orthopedic surgeon she knew—she just happened to have his phone number in her purse. "I never made such a desperate call in my life," says Donna. "I told him, 'If you don't come, my mother will die.'"

The new orthopedic surgeon didn't even need an X-ray to tell what was wrong with Madeline's hip, though he ordered one anyway to confirm his diagnosis. One of the 4-inch pins, about the size of a fountain pen, used to hold the broken hip bones in place had come loose and had migrated out of the bone and into the muscles surrounding her hip. No wonder every time Madeline moved she felt like a knife was poking her. The surgeon later told Madeline and Donna that the earlier X-ray clearly showed the problem, which should have been corrected. It was right there on the X-ray. But, Donna recalls, "He refused to put this in writing. He told me point-blank that the other doctors are his colleagues and he can't go against them." And he admitted that most of his work these days is fixing other physicians' mistakes, but said she shouldn't tell other physicians that he said this. Donna says, "It's a good-old-boys' network, and the state medical boards need to be reformed."

Madeline needed a second surgery to remove the pin and replace the fractured hip bone with a metal joint. It took her three years to recover her strength from her ordeal. Today, she walks with a permanent limp and wears special shoes to keep her back from hurting. "He ruined my life," Madeline says. "At seventy-five years of age, I spent from September sixth to December second in hospitals or rehabilitation centers recovering from a fractured hip that should have healed in six weeks. At this point, I do not know if I will ever be able to walk independently and without pain."

Donna says, "Even with all my knowledge as a nurse, I was basically ignored. It wasn't until I took the situation into my own hands and called the orthopedic surgeon that I knew things had turned around."

■ JUSTIN, STAR QUARTERBACK AND COLLEGE STUDENT

Even the healthiest among us can fall victim, rapidly, to a medical mistake. In Justin's case, several physicians overlooked a rampant infection that quickly killed the nineteen-year-old freshman. His troubles began with flu-like symptoms and pain in his right chest and shoulder area. A former star quarterback in high school, Justin was a tough young man, but his symptoms were rapidly getting worse, so he went to the emergency department at his local hospital with his mother, Carey. He spent the next seven and a half hours there while X-rays were taken but no blood work, despite the fact that his blood pressure was very low and his heart was beating at a rapid 120 beats per minute. The emergency room physician diagnosed his problem as a pinched nerve and sent him home with "enough pain medicine to kill an elephant," his mother recalls.

As the day progressed, Justin's condition remained the same. Carey called their family physician's office and reported to the nurse what had transpired at the ER and asked if anything else should be done. The nurse said she would relay this information to the doctor. "Justin spent a restless night and did not improve," his mother recalls. "The next morning he was extremely weak and this is when I knew he was getting worse." She called his doctor again and he dismissed her concerns, attributing Justin's reaction to the pain medications. Following her instincts as a mother, Carey says, "I called an ambulance and took Justin back to the ER where he was the day before." By the time Justin arrived, he was in shock. A massive infection caused by the same bacteria that killed Muppets creator Jim Henson—group A streptococcus bacteria—was shutting down Justin's major organs. Despite infusions of antibiotics, Justin died seven hours later, a victim, as his mother says, of a missed diagnosis and indifference.

From Anguish to Action

A farmer from New England, and a firsthand witness to harm caused by an incompetent doctor, wrote to us and said, "As a nation we cannot address the problem of medical errors until it can be accurately defined, and it cannot be defined until the closets are open." And so by telling the stories and giving the American people a chance to speak out on medical mistakes, only then can the closets be opened. Only then will light be shed on events that have remained in the shadows of our society.

As Daniel, the former White House staffer, wrote, "Perhaps my travail may become a torch to light a new way." All of these people who shared their stories are lighting a new way, channeling their anguish and grief into constructive action. Diana testified before Congress to let our nation's policymakers know about the scourge of medical mistakes. Rebecca lobbied vigorously for changes in state law that now allow a patient or family to file a complaint and see the results of the state health department's investigation. Amazingly, before this bill became law, neither the patient, the family, nor the general public had a right to review the findings of state investigations.

Three thousand miles across the country, Lewis's mom is lobbying her state legislature to enact a law that would require residents to wear identification that would notify patients and families that they are doctors in training and not veteran doctors. As she says, "Great tragedy leads you down paths you never imagined."

Meanwhile, Patti is working from the inside to make health care safer for her patients in the hospital outpatient clinic where she works. The state where she lives now requires nurses licensed in the state to take continuing education courses in patient safety, and she is working to develop a continuing education curriculum to further this effort.

Mary, the news anchor, says, "Despite the loss of so much, my life is richer now. Before I leave this earth, I want to make sure that the next generation of people in pain don't have it as bad." Mary has started a Web site with a regular column on pain, which she hopes will help others. There are many others out there just like her. Mary recalls the news report she did—before her own surgery—on cosmetic procedures gone awry. "The phone rang off the hook for twenty-one days," she recalls. How uncanny that the program would foretell her own future.

These brave souls are among those who have the most to gain from preventing medical mistakes because they live in the aftermath. They are among those who are the most motivated to make mistakes as rare as can be.

Nearly all of these people and their families share one other common experience: The doctors and others involved in the care provided never acknowledged what was one of the most profound, life-changing experiences in these peoples' lives. It's as if the medical mistakes they lived through—and what others died from—never happened. In their battles to have the health care system be accountable, they have been stopped by the powerful forces working to maintain the medical status quo. They have all come up against the wall of silence.

3 | A Million Deaths a Decade

When Michael's mother, Ilene, first heard about the IOM report and its national estimates of deaths from medical mistakes, she exclaimed, "It's true. This does happen and not just to me. I'm not crazy!" She realized that other Americans just like her have experienced medical mistakes firsthand but have no idea they are in the company of so many others. Nor do many Americans know that the estimates undercount the real scope of errors in the U.S. health system.

The Tip of the Iceberg

The number of people who die each year from preventable medical mistakes in hospitals is more than the number of Americans who died in the Korean and Vietnam wars combined (as reported by official Pentagon sources). With as many as 100,000 deaths a year, medical mistakes kill almost as many people as AIDS, breast cancer, and motor vehicle accidents combined. Put another way, about 275 Americans may be dying *every day* because of preventable mistakes in hospitals alone.

Over the course of a decade, the impact of medical mistakes is breathtaking. A million deaths a decade is unfathomable. Will a million more die in the first decade of the twenty-first century? The truth is that we will never know the answer to this question if the status quo remains as is.

How did the experts arrive at the national estimates of deaths from medical mistakes? Most of the information comes from researchers who reviewed the medical records of people who had been admitted to hospitals. The 1991 *New England Journal of Medicine* article was based on the medical records of more than 30,000 people who had been hospitalized in New York State. The IOM relied on this rigorous study and one other, which used a similar approach and reviewed 15,000 medical records of people who had been admitted to hospitals in Utah and Colorado. *Because there is no national reporting of serious medical mistakes that result in death or serious injury as they happen in real time, these are among the best sources of information that exist.* The IOM report concluded that between 44,000 and 98,000 deaths from medical mistakes occur each year among hospitalized patients.

Yet these numbers don't even begin to tell the whole story. By virtually all accounts, the estimates of medical mistakes noted in the IOM report are an undercount, which is why we use the higher range of the estimate—nearly 100,000 deaths annually. Only those mistakes recorded by a doctor in a patient's medical record were counted, and physicians document less than 30 percent of mistakes. In a survey of specialist physicians, 44 percent of them said they were either discouraged from reporting, or encouraged not to report, medical mistakes.[1]

The firsthand accounts of people and their families who have borne the consequences of mistakes tell the same story of missing information in medical records, with more flourish. According to family members, the problem is not just medical mistakes being undocumented in the medical record. Justin's mother described how her son's records were altered after he died to hide the fact that his blood pressure and pulse were dangerously high when he was sent home from the emergency department. She recalled, "We received an anonymous phone call encouraging us to get the hospital medical records before they were altered any more than they had been, and we did."

Other families report how different the official medical record is from the detailed journals they kept. A husband, whose wife of fifty-three years died as a result of a hospital-acquired infection in a facility that had inconceivably poor infection control, describes how he kept his own journal. He said, "Whatever they did, I wrote it down. Anyone who got near her, I got their names. After all the time my wife spent in the hospital, I had a record of the sixty-nine doctors who came close to her, not including the residents." The husband's journal contradicted a good deal of what was written in the medical record, and his accounts were so detailed and verifiable that they could not be brushed off. "That journal I kept helped to get them to settle with me," he says.

The estimates of deaths from preventable medical mistakes are an undercount for another reason. The numbers don't include deaths from mistakes made during surgeries performed in physicians' offices and freestanding outpatient surgery centers. The Florida Board of Medicine, for example, placed an unprecedented temporary moratorium in September 2000 on certain surgeries performed in doctors' offices. Five patients had died over five months while undergoing elective surgery, mostly cosmetic surgery. A member of the Florida Board of Medicine was quoted in *American Medical News* as saying, "These are patients who are otherwise healthy, just trying to look better, and they're getting knocked off." Some anesthesiologists said the ban was justified because the death rate for some office surgeries is up to one hundred times the number of anesthesia deaths in hospitals and ambulatory surgery settings.

Deaths and injuries from medical mistakes during surgery in physician offices and freestanding outpatient surgery centers—injuries such as those sustained by Mary, the television news anchor—are not tallied. Because of the large volume of surgery performed in these facilities, the lack of information about errors that occur is extraordinary. The American Society of Anesthesiologists estimates that in 2003, more than 17 million surgical procedures will be performed in these settings, almost double the 9 million surgical procedures that will be performed on people admitted to the hospital.

Medical mistakes that result in deaths in nursing homes and rehabilitation centers are not counted, either. If Madeline, the grandmother whose failed hip surgery was missed by the orthopedic surgeon, had died while she was in the rehabilitation facility, the death probably would have been recorded as just another old woman dying after breaking her hip, rather than as the result of a preventable medical mistake.

Nor do the estimates include deaths that occur from prescriptions that are incorrectly filled at drug stores. The *Washington Post* reported that a Virginia woman picked up a prescription for her five-year-old son who had a bed-wetting problem. The prescription was mistakenly filled at five times the dose prescribed by the boy's doctor. Unknowingly, the mother gave her son the medicine, and the next morning, she found him dead.

Medical mistakes that occur when people undergo kidney dialysis at dialysis facilities also are not counted. More than 230,000 Americans with kidney disease receive treatment in 3,000 facilities nationwide. Many of these patients are older Americans with complex medical conditions such as diabetes and hypertension. According to the Office of the Inspector General (OIG) in the U.S. Department of Health and Human Services, injuries or deaths resulting from the care provided to these patients are not systematically reported. The OIG described a dialysis patient who was exposed to the toxic disinfectant used to sterilize the dialysis equipment. In another instance, a patient received too much of a drug that caused prolonged bleeding.

In sum, virtually no information exists on deaths or injuries from preventable medical mistakes outside the confines of a hospital.

About eighteen months after the IOM issued its report, an article in the *Journal of the American Medical Association* claimed that the number of deaths per year from medical mistakes is lower than the Institute's estimates. The Institute responded by pointing out that the new study excluded people who were likely to die from their illness within a few months. It issued a statement saying that, "Even patients with life expectancy of less than three months are entitled to safe and effective care." While the exact number of deaths from preventable medical mistakes will never be known, leaders in the medical profession do not dispute that preventable deaths occur in significant numbers.

Since the estimates of medical mistakes are of deaths in the hospital, only a few of the people whose stories you read, including Ockie, Marion, and Lewis, would be counted in the nearly 100,000 deaths per year from medical mistakes, since they died while they were hospitalized.

Of the other people who have shared their stories—Daniel, Mary, Elizabeth, Susan, Diana, and Madeline—only some were hospitalized at the time the mistakes occurred, and they all lived to tell about their injury and disability. But virtually nothing is known about how many more people are just like them, nor how many fully recover, subsequently die, or live with significant disability. No notoriety accompanies the aftermath of a medical error. As Daniel pointedly notes, "If as a White House official I was mugged on the street and injured, it might be a story in the *Washington Post*. But because I was injured in the health care system, no one knows about it." Similarly, there are untold numbers of preventable near misses or accidents that were caught in time by vigilant health care professionals, patients, or families.

Reporting from Behind the Wall

Although national estimates of medical mistakes exist, it is very hard for people who are anticipating a hospital stay to know how safe their own hospital is. Hospitals themselves often don't know how many medical mistakes occur every day in their own facilities. Staff are afraid to report mistakes, and even if hospitals do track errors, they don't want the public to know the numbers.

In a rare look at medical errors inside a hospital, the *Philadelphia Inquirer* in September 1999 put a human face on medical mistakes. A hospital's records on medical mistakes typically are kept confidential for legal reasons, so it is hard to find out about them. But when a health system in Pennsylvania went bankrupt and was bought by a health care company, the company filed a public account of the medical mistakes reported at one of the hospitals it was buying. These mistakes occurred from 1989 through the first six months of 1998.

What were some of the 598 mistakes reported? A patient with epilepsy died, and another was partially paralyzed, after having brain hemorrhages while surgery was performed by young doctors in training, who were inexperienced and inadequately supervised. Doctors wrote a letter to the hospital administrator describing the unfortunate death of the patient because of mistakes made by unsupervised surgical residents. Eight patients needed a second operation to remove instruments, cotton, or sponges left inside their bodies. Another patient received the wrong type of blood in a transfusion after a car accident. Four patients died after they received the wrong medication, too much medication, or no medication.

From War Heroes to Medical Casualties

As a nation, we owe it to our veterans to ensure that the health care provided to them is as safe as it can be. But the medical centers and other health care facilities operated by the Veterans Health Administration of the U.S. Department of Veterans Affairs (VA) are not immune from medical mistakes. Veterans' facilities are funded by the federal government, and Congress periodically holds hearings to review the care provided to veterans. At a hearing in the U.S.

House of Representatives in 1997, a medical director of a veterans' hospital had to explain the deaths of five patients in nineteen months: "an American Legion post commander whose lung was pierced by a misplaced stomach tube; a Korean War veteran whose cancer went untreated for fourteen months; a man who died after a fall in a wheelchair; a patient with Alzheimer's who died after wandering away from a nursing home; and a dialysis patient." He told the following story of how the veteran on dialysis died.

A sixty-year-old man lost a massive amount of blood while on dialysis. A nurse connected the patient to the dialysis machine but was having trouble connecting one of the lines. She was interrupted by a phone call, and a dialysis technician remained with the patient. When the nurse returned to the bedside, a container that could hold two liters of blood was overflowing. The nurse failed to connect the line to the patient. When his condition deteriorated rapidly, an emergency team was called to try to save the patient. The nurse and technician knowingly withheld information from the emergency team about the huge loss of blood.

To its enormous credit, however, in recent years the Veterans Health Administration has taken some bold steps to prevent medical mistakes and help victims and family members cope.

An Equal Opportunity Event?

When Vice President Dick Cheney received treatment for his heart condition shortly after the 2000 election, you can be sure that the doctors and nurses were careful. If they mistakenly gave him the wrong medication, for example, the consequences would no doubt reverberate. But what happens to other people, especially people with limited financial resources or education? Are Americans of modest means more likely to experience medical mistakes than people with higher incomes? A recent study published in the journal *Pediatrics* found that children in higher-income families had higher rates of medical errors. One reason is that wealthier families have more elective surgery. No matter the frequency of error, when it does happen, people with limited means who have to pay the cost of the care needed to repair the mistakes are disproportionately burdened compared with those who are well insured and have a job to return to after they recover.

Burying Their Mistakes

Medical mistakes often go unreported in a patient's medical record, which makes it difficult to know how frequently they occur. Another way that medical mistakes are kept from view is that they are buried—literally. Autopsies can provide doctors and medical students with a firsthand look at disease and how it affects the human body, and they can also shed light on whether medical mistakes were made. But autopsies are virtually extinct. Doctors rarely perform autopsies anymore; they usually are reserved for deaths that result from criminal activity rather than disease. In the 1950s, autopsies were conducted on about 50 percent of people who died in hospitals; now the figure is only about 5 percent.

Why are so few autopsies conducted? Consider the parents of a newborn who told *60 Minutes* that a hospital allegedly covered up a big mistake when their baby died unexpectedly. The grieving parents asked for an autopsy, but the hospital staff discouraged them from making such a request. The parents sued the hospital because they thought it was hiding a delivery that had gone bad, and they settled with the hospital for an undisclosed amount.

Another reason autopsies are so rare is that hospitals have to pay for them out of overhead since they can't bill Medicare for them directly as they used to. Families who want to know the actual cause of death of their loved one will probably have to pay for an autopsy. Patient advocates recommend that an autopsy be conducted independent of the hospital where the patient died so there is no conflict of interest. But at a cost of $2,000 to $3,000, autopsies are out of reach for many people.

Public Perception of the Risks

Even without good information about the magnitude of medical mistakes, the public knows that health care is not as safe as it should be. A survey led by researchers at the Harvard School of Public Health found that 42 percent of people questioned believed they or a family member received care that involved medical mistakes.[2] Another survey conducted by the federal government's Agency for Healthcare Research and Quality and the Kaiser Family Foundation found that almost half of all Americans—47 percent—are very concerned that a serious mistake will be made when they receive health care services.[3]

How does the public perceive the risks of medical mistakes in health care as compared with other risks? Americans viewed health care as safer than a nuclear power plant, but less safe than airline travel or the workplace. In fact, this public perception is not too far off the mark. A report prepared for state policymakers in Massachusetts noted that the risk of dying while being a patient in a hospital in Massachusetts was 200 times greater than the risk of dying in a vehicular accident, and 2,000 times greater than the risk of being injured while working in a chemical plant or flying in an airplane.

Perceptions Behind the Wall

Conscientious doctors, nurses, and pharmacists working in health care are losing faith, too. They are issuing warnings from the front lines about the deteriorating "care" in health care. More than half of physicians surveyed reported that in the past five years, their ability to provide quality health care has deteriorated. Physicians who are leaders in their field, and who have spent their careers trying to improve the quality of patient care, are unable to make the system work safely and effectively even for themselves or their parents, spouses, or children. This is not just a case of bad care for the underprivileged. As Dr. Donald Berwick, a nationally recognized leader in improving the safety of health care, said in a speech to health care professionals at a national forum on quality improvement, "We are doing harm. We need to stop it."

Nurses are leaving their beloved profession in droves, especially hospital nurses, because they say they cannot safely take care of patients. They are overworked and overstressed. Nurses most concerned about their hospital cited preventable medical mistakes and complications after surgery as raising the greatest worry. *More than 40 percent of nurses say they would not recommend the hospital where they work to family members needing care.*

More Than Just a Human Cost

Medical mistakes exact a large human toll on people and their families, but there's another side to the story. All too often, medical mistakes leave a family in financial tatters. Of the 1.3 million Americans who file for personal bankruptcy each year, about 500,000 do so either because they are no longer able to work as a result of debilitating disease or injury and/or medical bills that spiraled out of control. Some of these bankruptcies are the result of costs that people and their families have to bear because of the inherent risks in the health system as well as mistakes.

A two-and-a-half-year-old boy named Daniel contracted HIV from contaminated blood he received during surgery shortly after he was born in 1984. This was before blood was screened for the virus, which was just emerging as a serious public health threat, so this would not count as a medical error. Yet the financial ramifications of this tragedy would prove insurmountable. Daniel's family was just about to move from California to Colorado when they were given the devastating news of his diagnosis. Before the move, both parents had quit their jobs, which provided them with good insurance coverage. When they arrived in Colorado and tried to buy private insurance, no insurance company would cover Daniel's preexisting condition.

With mounting bills for Daniel's care, the family had to file for personal bankruptcy. His mother, Linda, recalls, "When I was given the consent form to sign for Daniel's surgery, a little voice inside caused me to hesitate. But I went ahead anyway. In the consent form the hospital absolved itself of all responsibility for the blood supply. For years I blamed myself for signing that paper."

The state's Medicaid program, which provides health insurance coverage to families with limited financial means, seemed like a good choice to pay for Daniel's medical bills. While it offered a good safety net for the family, Linda says, "It was so demeaning to have to go on public assistance." When she got a job at a local hospital, she had private insurance coverage but it wouldn't cover Daniel, again because of his preexisting condition. In a no-win situation, Daniel lost his Medicaid coverage because his mom was now earning more money—but too much to meet the income eligibility criteria for the program. Linda had to leave her job anyway shortly thereafter to care for Daniel at home in his final days. He died just a few days shy of his sixteenth birthday.

In another instance reported in the journal *Inquiry*, a seventy-three-year-old woman had a heart attack and underwent cardiac catheterization, which helps doctors evaluate the condition of a patient's heart. In this procedure, a physician guides a catheter, or thin plastic tube, into a blood vessel in the arm or leg and into the heart. Immediately after the procedure, she suffered a hemorrhage from the catheter insertion site that resulted in a debilitating stroke. Physicians who reviewed her care concluded that the outcome was preventable and therefore a medical mistake. She spent forty-two days in the hospital and then was sent to a nursing home. Doctors estimated at the time that she would live for another twelve years, all of it in the nursing home, instead of at home. In total, the financial costs for her care were estimated at $607,335.[4] The human cost of being incapacitated and having to live in a nursing home for the rest of one's life cannot be measured in dollars and cents.

What is the total cost of medical mistakes, added up for all the people affected? While the human toll of medical mistakes is incalculable, the financial toll of preventable injuries resulting from medical mistakes is estimated by the IOM to cost $17 to $29 billion a year.

Paul O'Neill, former Secretary of the Treasury under President George W. Bush, put the cost of medical mistakes and poor-quality medical care in perspective. As the managing trustee of the Medicare trust fund while Treasury Secretary, O'Neill said that Medicare could save taxpayers' money by reducing medical mistakes and improving the overall quality of care. "If we could capture the potential that exists to do it right the first time, we'd probably reduce health and medical care costs 30 to 50 percent." Experts may differ on how accurate that estimate is, but the fact is that poor-quality health care costs a lot of money—and we're all paying for it.

The Firestorm Over Firestone

On August 9, 2000, the Bridgestone/Firestone Company announced that it was recalling 6.5 million tires, an event that was followed in May 2001 by an additional recall of 13 million tires by Ford Motor Company. These unprecedented corporate actions resulted from the firestorm that erupted over reports that approximately 200 people had died in accidents resulting from faulty Firestone tires. When the tires were linked to deaths and injuries, the news sent shock waves across the nation. Pictures of crashes caused by defective tires appeared on the nightly television news.

Almost immediately, Congress sprung into action. Corporate executives from Ford Motor Company and Bridgestone/Firestone appeared before Congress to be held publicly accountable, and members of Congress had harsh words for company executives for not acting quickly enough. The hearings started off with a news clip from a television station that put a human face on the deaths associated with the tires. Senator Richard Shelby, Chairman of the

Senate Transportation Subcommittee of the Senate Appropriations Committee, said, "I would like to know how it could take us ten years, dozens of lives, numerous lawsuits, substantial consumer complaints . . . before any action was taken to initiate an investigation into the safety of a product being used by millions of American families. Simply put, the American people deserve better." Officials of the National Highway Traffic Safety Administration were chided, too, by members of Congress for being asleep at the wheel. Two years earlier NHTSA had been told about the tread separation of the tires and the resulting roadway fatalities.

To quell fears among a worried public, Ford executives said that they planned to contact every owner of a Ford Explorer to show concern and make amends. Both companies had a vested interest in making things right because if they didn't, American consumers would exercise their right to take their business elsewhere. People would stop buying Ford Explorers and Bridgestone/Firestone tires. Millions, if not billions, of dollars were at stake, and the two companies took action to quell the public relations nightmare and, most importantly, prevent another needless death.

WHERE'S THE FIRESTORM OVER MEDICAL MISTAKES?

So what does the Bridgestone/Firestone debacle have to do with medical mistakes? Eight months earlier, in December 1999, the IOM report was released with estimates of the number of preventable deaths from medical mistakes. While widely covered in the media, there was no comparable outcry about the almost 100,000 deaths a year from medical mistakes. No one commented that it had been nearly a decade—and nearly a million deaths— since publication of the original study in the *New England Journal of Medicine* that had first identified the toll associated with medical mistakes. Congressional hearings were held but no health care executives were called on the carpet. No harsh words were exchanged, no one was scolded for inaction.

Why was the response by Congress to medical errors so muted and polite, compared with its response to the defective Bridgestone/Firestone tires? One reason might be that no federal agency tracks deaths and injuries from medical mistakes, as NHTSA tracks deaths and injuries from defective tires, or as the Occupational Safety and Health Administration monitors workplace accidents. Or it might be that deaths from defective tires are visible and can be shown on television news, while deaths from medical mistakes are not so obvious. In many cases, family members may not even know their loved one died from a medical mistake.

American society pays a great deal of deference to doctors, so much so that it may be politically incorrect to hold their actions up to public scrutiny. Their services may be needed someday, and no one wants to antagonize those who might be there to help when needed. In other instances, we may not really want to know what goes on because the reality could be too frightening.

Meanwhile, defenders of the status quo say that medical mistakes are inevitable because providing medical care today is complex. While it is true that humans will always make mistakes, this fact of life doesn't let the health care system off the hook. In fact, one health system CEO says he becomes "livid" when he hears that a hospital has a goal of reducing medical mistakes by 10 percent. He says, "Who would be satisfied if an airline had a goal of reducing the number of fatalities in air crashes by ten percent? It would be unacceptable."

Another reason for a light touch from Congress might be that no one is held accountable for mistakes in the health care system. There are few negative consequences to health care organizations that tolerate care that is not safe enough. This occurs even though the federal government pays—with taxpayer money—the bulk of the cost of medical mistakes through the Medicare program, since older Americans are more likely to experience medical mistakes. As a group, older Americans use the health care system more than others and are therefore more exposed to the possibility of error.

Members of Congress make decisions on how to allocate vast sums of our money for health care. They might use a light touch either because they don't know what to do, have a self-interest in maintaining the status quo, or don't have the political courage or muscle to face the special interests that benefit from the status quo. Yet medical mistakes don't discriminate; they affect Democrats, Republicans, and Independents alike.

Whatever the reason for the absence of a firestorm over medical errors—and the truth probably lies in all of these reasons—in the end, most of us Americans will be in a hospital someday as a patient, or require medical care that goes beyond "take two aspirin and call me in the morning." This is reason enough to do everything to make medical mistakes as rare as possible.

Among the people whose stories you have read here, there is little optimism that medical mistakes will be corrected anytime soon. Patients don't boycott hospitals or doctors, in an obvious fashion—at least not yet. But some people who have had a bad experience in health care quietly vow to stay away from doctors and hospitals as much as they can. One woman in her forties who, with her husband, has had a series of bad but not life-threatening experiences put it bluntly: "I won't go back." This is the only way they know to fight back—and protect themselves.

Hitting Rock Bottom over Mounting Numbers

Medical errors are like the stock market: sometimes things have to get really bad and hit rock bottom before they turn around and go up again. Have we hit rock bottom with medical mistakes? Probably not, and here's why.

Some hospitals with conscientious and capable leadership have made changes for the better. Dana-Farber Cancer Institute in Boston hit rock bottom in November 1994 when a patient named Betsy Lehman was given an overdose of chemotherapy that killed her. Bad publicity put the tragedy in the spotlight and the hospital in the hot seat. Many believe that if the patient hadn't been a well-known *Boston Globe* health reporter, the mistake would have never seen the light of day. To save itself and its reputation, the hospital had nowhere to go but up, and it has made substantial improvements to prevent mistakes.

But when medical mistakes happen outside the public eye, too little is done to find out what went wrong and prevent the next mistake. An enlightened former CEO of a large health system in the Midwest tells the story of when he gave a speech on the need for hospitals to reduce errors. A pharmacist who works in a hospital came up to him and said, "I wish you were the CEO where I work. Not long ago my CEO said to me, 'We need to get going on patient safety, and because you've been interested in this, I'd like you to take the lead on it.'" While this was no doubt a boost to the employee, he already had a full-time job.

Hospital patient safety must start at the top, with the CEO and the board; it can't be delegated to an employee. So, like many if not most hospitals, the one where this pharmacist works hasn't hit rock bottom yet. Only when it does will the hospital start to take error prevention seriously.

How Many More?

Throughout our history, Americans have shown we have the know-how, perseverance, and courage to correct many ills in our society. When tragedy strikes, volunteers from all walks of life come to do wondrous works of mercy. We fight for a cause when the stakes are high, whether it's civil rights, the environment, or the unmasking of the tobacco industry's deception, all of which illustrate the American people's capacity to demand that wrongs be corrected. Health care is next in line for redress.

Today, there is no organized national political constituency with the resources to vigorously advocate for those who have died or been injured by the health system. The adage that the squeaky wheel gets the grease applies to the cause at hand. The health care industry has not responded to the epidemic of medical mistakes in a way that any other sector of our economy would be compelled by the marketplace to do if nearly 100,000 people were dying every year because of preventable errors. If we don't start now, they'll keep coming—another million deaths in the next decade.

4 | What Is a Medical Mistake?

Errors in medicine have been made for as long as medicine has been practiced. The Greek medical texts, dating back to the time of Hippocrates, describe different kinds of errors. All pertain to the action of the physician rather than the "system," presumably because at that time there was no complex system of care as we have today. In his review of the Greek texts, Dr. Steven Miles, of the University of Minnesota, categorizes the reasons for physician error that were documented at that time: lack of technical skill, knowledge, and experience; overconfidence in an untested theory; desire to build a public reputation; among others.[1] One example of error he cites is as follows: "Tychon, at the siege of Datum, was struck in the chest by a catapult....The physician who removed the wood seemed...to leave the iron in at the diaphragm."[2]

Now, as then, preventable deaths and injuries happen at every stage of care from diagnosis and treatment to follow-up monitoring of the patient's condition after treatment. Here we describe different types of medical mistakes, illustrate them with the stories that you've already read, and introduce some new people. By no means is this a comprehensive list of the kinds of mistakes that occur, but it provides a way of categorizing them along the course of a patient's journey in the health system.

Missed Diagnosis

Making a correct diagnosis, particularly for some illnesses, can be a challenging stage in a patient's care, as diagnosis is often as much art as science. A missed diagnosis is a medical mistake when a physician does not perform an adequate diagnostic workup to determine the underlying cause of symptoms. Even with the best diagnostic workup, the correct synthesis of the findings is needed to come up with an accurate diagnosis. Getting to the right diagnosis is a process of discovery that often evolves over time as new information becomes known.

Here is how one doctor describes it: "If a woman comes in and reports difficulty breathing, I might be thinking viral pneumonia, with a small chance of a blood clot in the lung. The calculation changes when she says she just returned from a long flight from Europe, because blood clots can form while on long airplane trips. It changes further when she reports a history of sickle cell disease. Because a blood clot in the lung is a more serious diagnosis and requires more rapid intervention than a viral pneumonia, I will start an anticoagulant while we sort this out. So there are three kinds of potential errors: one is failing to ask the right questions and do the right tests to get the answer, one is failing to come to a working diagnosis in a timely way, and the third is failing to give certain kinds of therapy pending confirmation or elimination of a diagnosis."

Not every missed diagnosis is the result of error. Some patients have rare conditions that are simply unknowable even with today's diagnostic capability. Then there are patients who don't follow up on a doctor's recommendation to have a certain diagnostic test performed or to be examined by a specialist. In fact, to protect themselves from accusations of missed diagnoses, some doctors send patients letters by registered mail restating their recommendations. But jumping to conclusions without verifying an initial diagnosis can lead to medical mistakes.

• Justin, the nineteen-year-old college freshman, died when an emergency room physician misdiagnosed a rampant infection as a pinched nerve. He was sent home with a low blood pressure reading and very rapid pulse. His mom put it this way, "They didn't think out of the box. If they hear hoofbeats, they think horses. They don't think about zebras."

• Elizabeth, the eight-year-old who had survived kidney cancer, became paralyzed from the waist down after a recurrence of cancer was missed. Her mother says that if an MRI had been done three months earlier, when Elizabeth first began to complain about increasing pain, Elizabeth's tumor would have been diagnosed and probably would have responded to treatment, as it later did. Even if the MRI hadn't been ordered three months earlier, Elizabeth's deteriorating condition signaled warnings that should have been heeded.

• A middle-aged man went to his doctor for a checkup for rectal bleeding, as recounted in the 1991 *New England Journal of Medicine* article on medical mistakes. The doctor performed a limited sigmoidoscopy, a procedure that enables a physician to look at the inside of the large intestine, and the results were negative. The rectal bleeding continued, but the doctor reassured his patient. Nevertheless, the man started losing weight. Almost two years later, the patient had lost thirty pounds and was admitted to the hospital. He was diagnosed with colon cancer that had spread to his liver. A physician who conducted an independent review of the man's medical record concluded that if the condition had been properly diagnosed from the beginning, the cancer might have been curable.[3]

Delays in diagnosis can occur when professional and personal relationships among health care providers go sour. In other circumstances, the relationships might be on perfectly good terms, but when patients switch primary care doctors, or when primary care doctors consult with specialist physicians, the communication between doctors about the patient's condition might be exceedingly poor and the correct diagnosis can be missed.

• Diana, the former Air Force intelligence officer, had a dislocated hip that was left undiagnosed for six weeks. It was missed not because of an inadequate diagnostic workup but because her physician seemed to abandon her, a violation of fundamental medical ethics. Only afterward did she learn that her doctor had left the state directly after the surgery. "He went to Florida, where he maintained a second practice both because he liked to vacation there and because there are a lot of elderly people there who probably need joint replacements," she explains. "I didn't see him until six weeks after the surgery, and by then, my hip was in very bad shape. He had a falling-out with a former colleague who was a well-known orthopedic surgeon at the hospital I was transferred to, and my surgeon didn't want his former partner to have anything to do with me," Diana recollects. "He let his personal animosities get in the way of my care."

• A New England man, a retired pilot, had a primary care physician for many years who stopped seeing patients when he started a full-time administrative job in a nearby health care facility. A new primary care physician took over the man's care. Test results in his medical record showed warning signs for cancer but the new physician didn't follow up and neither had his long-standing primary care physician. The two doctors never discussed the man's condition. The man obtained his own medical record and reviewed it. He brought the test results to his doctor's attention. Only then were the follow-up tests performed that showed a definitive cancer diagnosis. Surgery was performed, and the former pilot is now cancer-free. His vigilance possibly saved his life.

Mistakes During Treatment

Even when a condition is diagnosed properly, different types of errors can occur in the complex course of treatment. Some are errors of omission, that is, care that should have been provided but was not. For patients who are correctly diagnosed with a heart attack, for example, an insufficient response to fluid management and control of arrhythmias is an error of omission that can contribute to patients' deaths. Other errors are errors of commission, or actions that are performed that lead to harm. Leaving foreign objects in a person during surgery is one such example.

• A Seattle man, Don, walked through airport security at Seattle-Tacoma Airport and the metal detector went off. He emptied his pockets of keys and change, and still it went off. Don was puzzled, but the security personnel waved him through. A few months earlier Don had had surgery to remove a very large cancerous tumor near his appendix and was in such excruciating pain afterward that he thought the cancer had returned. In fact, for several months he thought he was dying because the pain was so bad. After he returned from his trip, he went for a computerized tomography (CT) scan, which revealed that a thirteen-inch metal retractor had been left in him during the surgery. "I was just floored," he says, when asked his reaction to the news. "That thing was like the size of a lawn-mower blade. But all in all, I was relieved because at least I knew it wasn't the cancer coming back and I wasn't dying." He arranged to have a second surgery at another hospital to remove the metal object. The first hospital apologized and said that it planned to learn from this mistake. He says, "I hope that no one else will have to go through what I did."

• A patient at a hospital in New England was receiving oxygen, and the oxygen mask was attached to a tank of nitrous oxide instead of oxygen. She died. Shortly afterward, a second patient died from the same mistake at the same hospital. To its credit, the hospital took the unprecedented step of making the mistakes known to the public.

• A Connecticut woman went into a hospital for a coronary angioplasty, a procedure used to clear blockages in arteries that bring blood to the heart. She ended up having heart bypass surgery. She died from a hospital-acquired infection that was attributed to the hospital's exceedingly poor infection control practices. The hospital fought her husband all the way to the Supreme Court of the state of Connecticut to keep its internal records—which showed inattention to rampant infection—sealed. The hospital lost the case and had to open its infection records, which showed that at one point a significant percentage of other patients were similarly infected.

Errors in treatment also occur when doctors who are still in training are inadequately supervised while providing care to patients. Training programs are required to ensure that an experienced physician closely supervises residents, but this is not always the case. The results can be tragic when less-experienced doctors who are still in training get in over their heads.

• Marlene was in a New York hospital to deliver her third child and was under the care of the attending obstetrician. Her husband, Leonard, describes how an unsupervised resident came to administer an epidural without her consent and did so in a manner that resulted in his wife's death. Leonard recalls that if he and his wife had known that it was a resident who was performing the procedure, they would have requested an attending, or supervising, physician. "The resident delayed getting help because she was too busy trying to cover up her error," Marlene's husband says. The state health department promptly investigated the case at her husband's request and found the hospital to be in violation of the state hospital code. A baby girl was born who will never know her mother. Leonard mourns the loss of "my friend, my high school sweetheart, my soul mate, my bride."

• Young Lewis's obvious symptoms of internal bleeding were missed by numerous residents, and his mother's repeated requests that a veteran doctor examine her son were ignored. By the time an experienced physician saw the boy, he had lost too much blood to survive.

Medication Mistakes

Medication errors are some of the most common medical mistakes, in part because literally billions of doses of prescription drugs are administered every year. The process of prescribing, dispensing, and administering these doses is teeming with possibilities for error. Not all bad outcomes from medications are the result of errors, however. For instance, patients who don't know they are allergic to penicillin and are given it can go into anaphylactic shock, which is the severest form of an allergic reaction. Without immediate medical attention, anaphylactic shock can result in death. There is no way to diagnose an allergy to penicillin, and without foreknowledge of an allergy, no error occurs if penicillin is prescribed. On the other hand, it *does* qualify as an error if a patient is given penicillin when the medical record states that the patient is allergic to it. It is also an error if a patient is given penicillin and has an allergic reaction that the doctor does not diagnose and treat.

Here are just a few examples of medical mistakes involving prescription medicines.

• Sandy's dad received a refill for heparin, a drug used to prevent blood clots. Because the pharmacy made a mistake in refilling the prescription for heparin, it was only 10 percent of the strength he had been prescribed. He developed a blood clot in his lung and died.

• A seventy-three-year-old New Jersey man, John, was hospitalized for advanced prostate cancer. While John's wife and other family members were in the room, the nurse came to administer a drug through his intravenous line. Fortunately, his wife noticed that her husband was allergic to the drug about to be administered, a fact that was noted in his medical record but overlooked by the staff providing his care. She said to the nurse, "I think he's allergic to that drug." She saved her husband's life that day.

Inadequate Postoperative Care

The growth in outpatient surgery performed in physicians' offices and freestanding surgical centers—a relief to people who want to avoid an overnight stay in a hospital—offers little opportunity for careful monitoring at home in the days following surgery. The warning signs of complications can be more easily missed, although even when a patient is in the hospital, overworked staff may not monitor a patient as closely as necessary. Here are examples of horrifying outcomes that can result from inadequate post-surgical care.

• A healthy twenty-three-year-old woman in Florida had elective surgery to remove hemorrhoids. After returning home, she began having a great deal of pain and went to the hospital emergency department. She died shortly thereafter, reportedly from sepsis, a toxic condition resulting from infection. The family is devastated and wonders how their daughter could have died.

• Susan's experience with a laparoscopic procedure illustrates a physician's failure to heed warning signs of known complications. An astute patient, with the support of friends taking care of her, she sought medical attention that saved her life.

Mistaken Identity

In this day and age when identity checks are becoming the norm in society generally, and when technology to verify a person's identity is advancing with great sophistication, it seems hard to imagine how the identity of two patients in a hospital can be mixed up. Nevertheless, patients do end up in the wrong bed or identified with the wrong test results because of human error.

• A Maryland woman describes the following scene in the hospital. "My husband was admitted to the hospital, and when he was brought back to his room after surgery, his roommate was gone and the nurse insisted on putting my husband in his roommate's bed. I equally insisted that she was wrong, that it wasn't his bed. She was emphatic, and so I became more emphatic. He finally got in the right bed. Imagine if I hadn't been there? Both my husband and his roommate could have suffered something really bad."

• A sixty-year-old veteran with cancer of the esophagus had surgery. He suffered complications and had a second operation. While on the operating table, he received two units of blood meant for another patient. He suffered cardiac arrest and died. An autopsy found that he died from an incompatible blood transfusion. The blood he received was for another patient who had had surgery in the same operating room just before he did. The blood intended for the veteran was in another operating room. Before the blood was transfused, no one verified the patient's identity by looking at his wristband to see if it matched the name on the two units of blood.

• A Wisconsin woman was diagnosed with breast cancer in both of her breasts. She underwent a double mastectomy to remove the cancerous breasts. Later, her doctors realized that the cancer diagnosis was a mistake. Her biopsy results had been mixed up with someone else's. The woman never had cancer.

In some instances, a surgeon may perform the wrong procedure on a patient because the identity of the patient wasn't verified before the procedure was started.

• A Florida surgeon mistakenly removed the left breast of a woman who was to have only a lumpectomy. How did this happen? Two women were awaiting surgery and the doctor asked that the patient scheduled for the mastectomy be brought into the operating room. Hospital staff wheeled in the wrong patient. After the surgeon removed the woman's breast, another doctor realized that the woman still waiting for surgery was the patient who was to have her breast removed. According to the Associated Press, the Florida Medical Board dealt with twenty instances in the year 2000 when patients had undergone procedures meant for another patient. It's unknown whether this number is an undercount.

In other instances, a surgeon might perform the wrong surgery on the right patient.

• One of the medical mistakes reported in the *Philadelphia Inquirer* in September 1999 happened to a seventy-nine-year-old man who was to have a procedure performed on his left lung, but his right lung was operated on instead.

• In December 2001, the Joint Commission on the Accreditation of Healthcare Organizations (JCAHO), the entity that accredits health care facilities, identified examples of surgical mistakes that health care professionals reported to them: a patient had the wrong hip joint replaced, a biopsy was conducted on the wrong side of a patient's brain, a patient had the wrong spinal disk fused, and another had a healthy kidney removed instead of a cancerous one.

The Limits of What Is Possible

While reading about these different types of medical mistakes, it would be wrong to conclude that every bad outcome from medical treatment is a mistake. Patients can have bad outcomes that are not the result of substandard care but the inevitable consequences of the progression of a disease or condition, or of treatment that is the best effort of skilled and knowledgeable doctors and nurses.

Expectations for what medicine can accomplish may sometimes be unrealistically high, especially in a country where the frontier of science and medicine is expanding at a faster pace than ever. Both doctors and patients would do well to be humbled by the observations of Dr. Lewis Thomas, a former dean of Yale Medical School and former president of Memorial Sloan-Kettering Cancer Center in New York, who said in his book, *The Fragile Species,* "The trouble with medicine today is that we simply do not know enough, we are still a largely ignorant profession, faced by an array of illnesses that we do not really understand, unable to do much beyond trying to make the right diagnosis, shoring things up whenever we can."[4] Within these limits of human endeavor, the task at hand is to do the best with the knowledge that exists and as carefully as possible. When medicine doesn't use what *is* known, mistakes occur and people are harmed.

Errors Repeat Themselves

While many patients and families can understand that doctors and nurses will make mistakes, they have zero tolerance for the idea that the error will not be used to improve medical practice, as the ancient Greeks said it should be. As Dr. Miles notes, Greek medical texts highlighted the importance of physicians sharing information among themselves about medical errors as a way of improving medical practice. Too often, though, this sharing of information about error does not occur, and many of the same types of mistakes—in diagnosis, treatment, and follow-up care—are repeated over and over again.

Meanwhile, the medical profession has demonstrated an inability to weed out its members whose track records of repeated errors suggest they should not be entrusted with the privilege of having a license to practice medicine. In other cases, physicians might be quite competent performing certain procedures but are tempted to try their hand at other procedures they are not sufficiently knowledgeable or skilled to perform, a problem that dates back to the ancient Greeks.

Errors are bound to be repeated when competent professionals don't use techniques that have been proven to reduce mistakes. The American Academy of Orthopedic Surgeons started a "Sign Your Site" program in 1997 that encouraged surgeons to mark the site of surgery in advance with a permanent marker. If a patient is planning to have knee surgery on the right knee, the surgeon should mark that knee in advance and mark a "No" on the left knee. The patient should make sure to ask if it is not done. But only about 60 percent of orthopedic surgeons comply with these recommendations. The president of JCAHO, Dr. Dennis O'Leary, said, "The know-how to create systems that prevent wrong-site surgeries has existed for years, yet the number of errors has not decreased." So why are recommended techniques to reduce preventable medical mistakes not used and the same errors made over and over again? Why have health care facilities—whose purpose is to heal and which should have the greatest motivation to prevent harm—not adopted practices that reduce the likelihood of mistakes?

Part of the answer is complacency. If wrong-site surgeries are never tallied and tracked over time, by hospital where they occur and by physician who made the mistake, then there is no appreciation for how often and where they occur. Without this information, the problem doesn't rise to the top of all the other crises that hospital administrators and doctors have to manage. Adding to the complacency is an exaggerated form of confidence that says, "That will never happen on my watch."

Another contributing factor is that health care professionals and administrators do not have, and were never taught, the knowledge and skills needed to put systems in place that make the right thing to do—in this case, sign the site of surgery in advance—the default course of action. Right now, it is an option. When pilots prepare for takeoff, they read the checklist out loud even though they probably know it by heart. It doesn't matter. It is not an option to overlook key safety checks before takeoff. Safety is an integral part of pilot training, and shortcuts can lead to disaster.

Albert Einstein once said, "We can't solve problems by using the same kind of thinking we used when we created them." To make medical mistakes as rare as possible, new knowledge and skills are needed in health care organizations. Without new ways of thinking and doing, it is exceedingly difficult to create an environment in health care where the safety of patients is the top priority. To illustrate this point, we heard about a conversation with a hospital CEO who was asked how she knew when a medical error occurred in her hospital. She replied that she knew when a mistake had happened whenever a nurse was fired. Sadly, this approach illustrates how little knowledge this CEO has about the root causes of medical mistakes and effective solutions to prevent them. Most medical mistakes occur because doctors, nurses, pharmacists, and other health care professionals work in health care organizations that are not designed to weed out the possibility of error. Just as automobiles are designed so they cannot start in drive or reverse and cause accidents, health care facilities need to be designed to minimize mistakes.

Learning from Mistakes

Recognizing the need to look to other industries for answers on how to prevent mistakes, the IOM panel spent some time learning about why mistakes occur in industries that are known to be high risk, such as the airline and nuclear power industries, and how mistakes are prevented. These industries have been highly successful in designing organizations and processes that minimize the chance that a mistake will occur—or, if it does, that it is caught in time and triggers a response that requires corrective action.

The accidents that befell NASA space shuttles *Challenger* and *Columbia* have relevance to health care because they occurred as a result of a sequence of events that added up and led to disaster. (At this writing, the exact cause of the *Columbia* tragedy is being investigated by authorities.) Analyzing such events is a constructive way to understand how mistakes occur and to learn how to prevent a chain of events from unraveling. As with other industries, health care is a complex enterprise involving many moving parts and people. While humans will inevitably make mistakes, the key is to put systems and procedures in place that prevent them.

Here is a very simple example. In February 1998, JCAHO issued an alert to health care providers in response to hospital reports it was receiving that patients were dying as a result of errors in the administration of potassium chloride, a chemical commonly used in health care. Patients were being given concentrated solutions of potassium chloride by mistake, which led to their deaths. JCAHO recommended a simple answer to this problem: hospitals should remove all concentrated solutions of potassium chloride from the stocks on nursing units. The result? It is receiving fewer reports of deaths from concentrations of potassium chloride, a hopeful sign. But how long has this problem existed and why did it take so long to fix it? And at what cost in lost lives?

The more fundamental question is why the health care industry is a laggard compared with other sectors in employing state-of-the-art practices to make human error as rare as possible. The answer is it has had little incentive to do so. Failures in airline and nuclear power plant safety are highly publicized events, and the public demands accountability from these industries. In contrast, medical mistakes are less obvious. They happen one at a time, and when they do happen they traditionally have been swept under the rug. Some doctors say that in medical school they were taught that they would make mistakes and they would "have to learn to bury them."

When the culture of a profession for many years has been to bury its mistakes, it is not surprising that health care doesn't learn from its mistakes and makes the same ones over and over again. Alexander Pope, the eighteenth-century English poet, once said, "To err is human, to forgive divine." The title of the IOM report, "*To Err Is Human*," is apropos because as humans, we all make mistakes. But if we don't learn from mistakes, make no efforts to prevent them, and continue to make them, we are guilty of a far greater mistake, and forgiveness is not always divine.

part two

Why Do Medical Mistakes Happen?

5 | Breeding Grounds for Error

Why do so many medical mistakes occur? A major reason is that hospitals and other health care facilities are breeding grounds for many different kinds of errors. Some poorly organized health care facilities don't ensure that their health care providers have the most current medical record for a patient they are about to examine. Others don't have systems in place to ensure that their doctors obtain the results of X-rays or CT scans they order. Breakdowns such as these happen every day, and in many cases it's not rocket science to fix them.

Yet they don't get fixed, and patients and families bear the result. So, too, do conscientious doctors, nurses, pharmacists, and others who endeavor to protect their patients as parents protect their young. Meanwhile, young doctors still in training are "raised" in this chaotic environment, often in an overworked and sleep-deprived state. They are never trained to work together with the other health care professionals, namely nurses, pharmacists, social workers, and physical therapists with whom they will work side by side, caring for patients for many years to come.

Most of the time, when medical errors occur, they are treated as isolated, individual events, rather than as a sign of a much larger underlying problem. Doctors, nurses, and others are sometimes forced to improvise to protect their own patients. But dealing with these problems one at a time is not effective.

"Unsafe acts are like mosquitoes," says James T. Reason, an expert on human error. "You can try to swat them one at a time, but there will always be others to take their place. The only effective remedy is to drain the swamps in which they breed."[1] With respect to medical mistakes, these "swamps" are organizations that are designed without safety in mind. They are characterized by overworked staff, poor communication among people taking care of the same patient, mistakes by individual providers, and budget pressures that force doctors, nurses, and administrators to cut corners.

■ A CASE OF MISSING MEDICAL RECORDS

A nurse practitioner shares her experience in being unable to access the inpatient medical records of patients whom she is now caring for at the outpatient clinic where she works. Here's what she says about how she tried for six months to have her health care facility change its systems but was unsuccessful and as a result, made a preventable medication mistake.

"Unwittingly, unknowingly, I based my decision regarding prescription dosages for a medication for a patient on outdated, inaccurate, and incomplete chart information. The previous two appointments this patient had were inpatient admissions to our hospital and those records were not in the chart that was given to me. I only had records from the time prior to his last two hospital stays. I had no way of knowing that I was not using up-to-date records, and I had no way of knowing that when I continued to prescribe the patient what I believed to be the current medication dose, I was actually now doubling the dose of the meds. While the patient was hospitalized on those two occasions, the dose was cut in half, but this was unknown to me. Thank goodness this patient was not harmed by our preventable errors."

She knew that this mistake was waiting to happen because of unsafe practices in the system where she works. She goes on to say, "I have been begging and pleading to try to get someone to listen to the real problem that exists with our medical records processes which place my patients at risk for preventable medication errors every day. For many months now, the medical records managers have said that they do not have time to deal with what they consider to be my problem to solve, as they have no way of knowing if my scheduled patients have been in our hospital or not.

"Having little success, I stated that I would no longer see patients for scheduled appointments without having their records on my desk at the time of the patients' appointments. Shortly thereafter, the medical records coordinator finally said she might begin having medical records staff check the computer for recent hospital admissions when screening my patient charts prior to scheduled appointments. I hope for more scraps of concessions like this so that maybe my patients may receive safer care at that clinic."

In a letter to the CEO of the health care facility where she works, she describes her fruitless efforts. "My efforts to try and work towards resolving the longstanding medical records policy and procedure problems that have led to medical errors have been largely unsuccessful. I don't know how else I can help resolve these problems so that I can, at a minimum, practice safely. I love my job and I truly enjoy working with my colleagues. But I need to be able to just do my job, with all its responsibilities and challenges, in the little time frame I am granted to do it in. Imagine that it was your family who was about to get their wrong and potentially injurious or lethal dose of medication, just because the system had a very longstanding, entrenched medical records system that prioritized something other than the safety of the patients."

Health care professionals all over the country walk this same tightrope every day, and if they fall off, it can have devastating consequences for them as well as for their patients. "If I made an error and ended up in court as a result of patient injury or death," she goes on to say, "I know that the judge will not feel any sympathy for me if I tell him or her that it wasn't my fault because my employer refused to give me the complete record while evaluating the patient. The judge will likely find that the error was preventable and that I was responsible for not reviewing all available records when making my decision to prescribe that medication, which was documented earlier in the record to have had an adverse reaction at that high a dose, and that I was professionally obligated to have accessed and reviewed that information. As licensed health care professionals, we are legally obligated to review previous available records, such as lab results, allergies, medication records, management notes, and consultant reports that are relevant to our decision making."

Because of direct intervention by the hospital's CEO, the policies and procedures regarding access to inpatient medical records finally changed, resulting in what this nurse practitioner describes to the CEO of the facility as "a positive and measurable change, with medical staff now being able to access and review appropriate patient medical records during scheduled appointments. For your interventions that have improved patient safety, I am very grateful."

Not to negate the small gains made, a lesson learned is that bad habits don't die quickly, and without continuous reinforcement, they resurface. Within six to nine months after the CEO stepped in to change the long-standing bad habits, the nurse practitioner still does not always have the necessary records for her appointments with her patients. "I guess I should just be grateful that I was able to protect my patients from preventable harm for that short six-month period of time," she says. "Again I'm sending letters to the risk manager, talking to the medical director and clinical and administrative managers of the hospital again, though it has become increasingly discouraging and disheartening."

■ A CASE OF RADIOLOGY TESTS POORLY CONDUCTED

Under pressure to read many poorly performed X-rays, CT scans, and ultrasounds conducted by inexperienced technicians, an exasperated radiologist writes, "I am deeply saddened by the quality of studies put out by most of the hospitals and private facilities. The radiologists are stressed out by being required to read more and more X-rays. To swim through the ocean of substandard work and emerge with needed information for the patient and consulting physicians has become a losing battle. I have found mistakes committed due to the rapidity with which the cases have to be read.

"This raises ethical issues and causes physical exhaustion that has reached a breaking point for several radiologists I know, including myself. Radiology is being used solely for the purpose of business, compromising standards, ethics, and patients' lives. Conscientious radiologists are unfairly victimized by escalating malpractice premiums due to the greed of others, yet I am extremely scared to speak out, for fear that if I do, I will not be able to get a job as a radiologist. My intentions are only to enforce quality and standards of care—just like I was taught during residency—and make my humble contribution to society."

■ A CASE OF THE MISSING CT SCAN REPORT

A conscientious physician shared the following story of a system failure encountered when caring for an elderly man. "I sent a patient for a head CT scan but never received a mail or fax copy of the CT scan report because of some kind of administrative snafu in radiology. I later found out it had shown a small benign tumor. Another CT scan four years later showed that the tumor had grown a lot in size and needed to be removed. Neither myself nor another doctor caring for the patient was tracking the tumor because we never saw the original report. Fortunately, the patient did fine.

"The problem was that there was no system to assure that every test ordered had a result that was seen and acknowledged by the ordering doctor. Depending on the doctor's memory to assure that every test result is seen and reviewed is obviously foolish. This is another example of a system problem. As a result of this incident I have set up a personal, handwritten tracking system for every single test that I order, and I check them off as the results come in."

■ **A CASE OF A NEVER-ORDERED CT SCAN**

An eighty-two-year-old man who smoked cigarettes for sixty years developed chronic obstructive pulmonary disease. The journal *American Family Physician* published an article that describes how the system failed him.[2] He was admitted to the hospital and had a chest X-ray, which found a small mass on his lungs. The resident wrote in his record a recommendation that the patient get a CT scan after discharge from the hospital to see what this mass might be.

About a month later the patient came to the clinic, and the resident remembered the patient but couldn't remember the medications he was taking and neither could the patient. Meanwhile, the hospital discharge records and radiology reports were at the hospital, not the clinic. The resident contacted the senior resident from the previous month, who remembered the patient and his medications. Thinking he had all the details, the resident didn't obtain or review the hospital reports.

Over time, the man's disease worsened. He came back to the clinic almost a year later, and a second chest X-ray showed a large lesion on his lung, later confirmed by a CT scan. The resident didn't remember that he had seen a lesion on the chest X-ray the previous year, so he went to the hospital to review the patient's record. He found the note he had written that stated that a CT scan would be obtained. The scan was never ordered; it "fell through the cracks." The patient died five months later.

■ CASES OF MISCOMMUNICATION

A physician describes how one patient bore the devastating consequences of miscommunication. "I had been taking care of a patient for several years who had been hospitalized. When I discharged him, I sent him home on a medication, and 'the wheels came off.' He was to be followed up in the clinic in a few days, but he was discharged in the evening after the clerk in the clinic had gone home, so he left the hospital without an appointment. He thought he was supposed to get one in the mail, and when he didn't, he thought he no longer needed any follow-up.

"While he was home, he started taking anti-inflammatory drugs for arthritis that he had been prescribed a long time ago, and aspirin. I wasn't aware of this—and both of these medications can interfere with the medication I had prescribed.

"He called the clinic on Friday and requested to talk to me, but I was busy seeing other patients, so he left a message with the clerk saying he felt dizzy. The clerk was sitting in for the regular staff person and was supposed to follow standard procedure and give a nurse this information. Instead, the clerk put the message in my mailbox that afternoon. Friday was my last day before a two-week vacation, and the message sat in my mailbox the whole time.

"When I returned from vacation I was shocked when I learned that about three days after he called and left a message for me, he was admitted to the hospital with a massive gastrointestinal bleed from an ulcer. The bleeding couldn't be stopped and most of his stomach had to be removed. During surgery, he needed sixteen units of blood.

"I immediately went to the medical floor and he had just been discharged. The nurses said he was 'enraged' by what had happened. I called him at home and asked him how he was. He was very cold and said, 'I almost died. I left a message for you and you never called back.'

"It was devastating. I wanted to see him face to face and asked him to come in. He looked horrible and was understandably very angry. He asked, 'What happened?' I explained about the drug interactions and the miscommunication, and started to cry. I said I was so very sorry, and then he started crying. 'Where are we going to go from here?' I asked. He's still my patient. It's distressing that as a physician, there is so much you can't control."

All too often, children, too, get caught in the snarled lines of communication among health care workers. Josie was an eighteen-month-old girl with big brown eyes who had just learned to say "I love you." She was admitted to a prestigious hospital on the East Coast after having suffered burns when she climbed into a hot bath. Her mother, Sorrel, had kept a day-and-night vigil at her bedside.

While in the hospital, Josie had become severely dehydrated, and Sorrel heard the doctor say that no more pain medications should be administered. Not long after that, a nurse came to administer more of the pain medication to Josie. Sorrel said to the nurse, "What are you doing?? There's an order for no more narcotics." The nurse said the orders had been changed and she administered the medication as planned.

Josie's mom recalls what happened fifteen minutes later. "Josie's heart stopped as I was rubbing her feet. She suffered cardiac arrest as a result of the dehydration and medication. Her eyes were fixed and I screamed for help. I stood helpless as a crowd of doctors and nurses came running into her room to resuscitate her. I was ushered into a small room with a chaplain, and the next time I saw Josie she had been moved back up to the pediatric intensive care unit. Doctors and nurses were standing around her bed. Josie was hooked up to many machines, and her leg was black and blue. I looked into their faces and said to them, '*You* did this to her, *NOW* you must fix her.' I was told to pray."

"Two days later," Sorrel writes, "Josie was taken off of life support. She died in our arms on a snowy night in what's considered to be one of the best hospitals in the world. Our lives were shattered and changed forever. Josie died from severe dehydration and misused narcotics. Careless human errors," she says. "It was a complete system breakdown. There was no communication between the doctors and the nurses, and they didn't listen to us—her parents."

Sorrel says she realizes now that, "What happened to us wasn't just a strike of lightning. There are thousands more people who die every year. I will not rest until we make something good come from her senseless death."

In a tragedy that garnered the attention of the nation, seventeen-year-old Jesica Santillan died after a heart and lungs of the wrong blood type were mistakenly implanted in her chest. Miscommunication between the transplant team and the organ donor service led each party to assume that the other had verified that the organs destined for transplant into Jesica correctly matched her blood type. The error was discovered while Jesica was still in the operating room; her immune system immediately began to attack the new heart and lungs as if they were harmful because the organs were different from her blood type. Six days later, a second transplant operation was performed with a new set of correctly matched heart and lungs. But two days after that, Jesica's doctors declared that her brain was no longer functioning, and she was removed from life support. Jesica's family, and the nation, were stunned.

■ A CASE OF MISTAKEN IDENTITY

The Annals of Internal Medicine described how a sixty-seven-year-old woman who went to a teaching hospital for a medical procedure was mistakenly identified as another patient.[3] Joan Morris (a pseudonym used to protect the identity of the patient) had fallen recently, and an MRI revealed that she had two large cerebral aneurysms that could cause a debilitating or even lethal stroke if they ruptured. The day after she was admitted to the hospital, her surgeon successfully treated one of the aneurysms; the other would require surgery in a future hospital stay. Joan was sent back to a room in the oncology unit instead of her original bed in a different unit and was expecting to go home the next day.

The next morning at 6:30 A.M. she found herself being wheeled into a room to have a test performed on her heart. About an hour into the procedure, Joan's physician turned up on the ward. He wanted to know where his patient was and was told she had been taken to the electrophysiology laboratory for a procedure. Only when he called the lab and asked why his patient was there did the mix-up become apparent, and the physician performing the procedure finally checked Joan's chart and realized the mistake.

How did this happen? Joan Morris was confused with seventy-seven-year-old Jane Morrison, who had been admitted to the hospital on the same day Joan arrived. Jane was scheduled to have a procedure to check her heart. A string of failures resulted in Joan being taken to have a procedure—despite her protests—even though no written orders for the procedure were in her chart, or a signed consent form. Before starting the procedure, the physician did not greet the patient or confirm her identity; her face was hidden by surgical drapes. A nurse present during the procedure mentioned that no patient named "Morris" was on the schedule, but the doctor told her this was the right patient. Joan recovered with no ill effects.

The Many Tribes in Health Care

The previous examples show how seemingly core functions in a hospital can go wrong, with the result that patients are put in harm's way, often despite the efforts of people who are trying their best to care for them. Yet even if all the day-to-day operations of a health care facility work smoothly, there's another characteristic of health care that nourishes it as a breeding ground for mistakes.

"Can you imagine a nurse yelling, 'Doctor, stop!' or even asking, 'Are you sure you want to do that?' No, you can't, and that needs to change," says Dr. Kenneth Kizer, a board-certified surgeon and president of the National Quality Forum, a Washington, D.C.-based nonprofit group.[4] The people who provide health care to patients are organized in different tribes. Doctors make up one tribe. Nurses constitute another tribe. Pharmacists, social workers, and technicians are all in separate tribes. These tribes are organized in a pecking order, with the doctors at the top of the pack, followed by each tribe with its own pecking order.

Members of these health care tribes are rarely, if ever, trained together while they are in medical, nursing, or pharmacy school, even though they will work side by side taking care of patients once they graduate. After that, virtually no training exists to help them learn how to work together, so instead of learning to understand and respect one another's role, there are chasms among the tribes. These chasms can result in errors, especially when professionals from different tribes are treating the same patient.

When decisions have to be made under great stress and with limited information, the tribal order can be a barrier to providing the highest-quality care. Gordon Sprenger is a former CEO of a health care system. Here's what he wrote in the *American Journal of Health-System Pharmacists* about the importance of teamwork. "I am reminded of an experience I had discussing landings on an aircraft carrier with a group of physicians. I was explaining that there was something different during these high-risk events that we can learn from. A surgeon in the group interrupted me, saying, 'The important factor is that there is a well-known leader—the ship's captain—who can call the shots.' What a teachable moment I had as we went on to discuss how the chain of command is suspended during landings. Any team member can stop a landing. The team is trained to communicate effectively with each other and to bring the plane safely in, and the team members share responsibility for that outcome."[5]

Teamwork Among Tribes

Diana, the former Air Force intelligence officer, could tell the difference between the hospital that cared for her competently and fostered a culture of teamwork, safety, accountability, and continuous improvement, and the hospital that could not even properly staff its facility with people who had the knowledge and skill to provide her with even the most basic care she needed. In her case, her surgeon wasn't even around for six weeks. It's hard to have a team if the players aren't trained or if they don't show up.

Here's what she says about the good teamwork she saw in action at the hospital that provided her with quality care. "Each staff member, at every level of responsibility, was competent, compassionate, skilled, and safety-conscious. Communications were open and ongoing among doctors, nurses, and technicians, and always included the patient as a respected, participating member of the team."

Just as naval aviators undergo air crew coordination training with all the other personnel who are involved in landing a jet on a moving ship as a way to prevent aviation mishaps, health care professionals need to do the same. Unfortunately, very few do. In some health care organizations, teams of health professionals are volunteering to be trained so they can work together better, especially in crisis situations when patients' lives are at risk, such as when a patient is hemorrhaging on the operating table. But for now, at least, this team training is the exception and far from the rule. Health care now has a lot of experts, but there are too few expert teams.

Inside the Health Care Cockpit

Imagine boarding a plane for a flight over the Atlantic and realizing that inside the cockpit, the captain, first officer, and flight engineer do not communicate very well. Imagine further that the flight crew has flown together before and the younger first officer is intimidated by his senior colleagues. He hesitates to speak up when the captain is about to make a mistake.

Many airline accidents are caused by breakdowns in communication, not technical failure. When a Korean Airlines flight crashed in Guam on August 6, 1997, two hundred and twenty-eight people were killed. The investigation by the National Transportation Safety Board found the cause: the first officer and flight engineer did not challenge a fatigued captain's failure to properly execute the approach to the airport.

Here in the United States, a first officer's deference to a flight captain was a factor that caused a Continental Airlines plane to land in Houston, Texas, in February 1996 without the landing gear extended. This is called a "wheels-up landing." The first officer tried to get the captain to abort the landing, but out of deference, did not challenge the captain's decision to continue the landing approach because he was afraid his own career would be jeopardized. Fortunately, no one died as a result of this failure in airline safety, but the plane's fuselage was severely damaged and the plane had to be scrapped.

These events are exceptions to an otherwise well-designed system that encourages good communication among the many professionals who pilot, service, and monitor our nation's passenger aircraft. Passengers can feel safe knowing that airline crews undergo intensive training in teamwork and communication. Junior pilots are taught that it is their duty to report mistakes and near misses, including those made by the senior pilot. This teamwork in the cockpit reduces the chances that a pilot will make a deadly error, or that a chain of mistakes will unfold. When errors do occur and planes crash, the National Transportation Safety Board examines every possible detail to understand and find the root causes of a crash. This very detailed information is fed back to the airlines, pilots, accident investigators, and the public to reduce the odds of the same error happening again. No system is perfect, and neither are humans. But in the airline industry, there is a big incentive to make flying as safe as possible. If a plane goes down, the pilots and crew go with it.

Health care has entirely different rules and bad habits that cause mistakes to occur and hinder learning from mistakes that do happen. In hospitals, many health care professionals move in and out of the health care cockpit, not just at cruising altitude but also at critical times that are equivalent to takeoff and landing. Doctors often lack complete information about the patients they are coming to see, including their medical history and the medicines they are taking. Nurses say that doctors do not always read the patient's medical chart. A doctor examining a patient may not know what a different doctor who came in previously said to the patient and family. In fact, patients describe instances in which two doctors gave completely contradictory information about their diagnosis and prognosis within the span of a few hours.

Doctors' views on teamwork are very different from those of airline pilots. When pilots, doctors, and nurses from the United States and other countries were surveyed, they were asked whether they agreed or disagreed with the statement that "junior members of the team should not question decisions made by more senior team members." Three percent of pilots agreed with that statement, but only 45 percent of surgeons agreed. Surgeons also were asked whether high levels of teamwork occur in their operating room. Sixty-four percent said yes, but only 28 percent of surgical nurses and 39 percent of anesthesiologists said yes.[6]

A story in USA Today described the tragic effects of miscommunication and poor teamwork. An eighteen-year-old boy came to the emergency room with symptoms of the flu. A doctor examined him, and he was sent home. He returned the next day by ambulance. He had meningitis, an inflammation of the lining of the brain. He died later that day. A nurse reflected on the event and acknowledged that she thought he had meningitis when he first came to the emergency room. She did not speak up because a few weeks earlier, a doctor had reprimanded her for saying something about the care of another patient. He had told her, "I'm the doctor, and you stick to nursing."[7]

The pecking order in the medical profession can clearly get in the way of good care for patients. In Lewis's case (the fifteen-year-old boy who died from internal bleeding from a perforated ulcer), the young resident overseeing his care felt so offended when Lewis's mom, Helen, insisted that a veteran doctor, an attending physician, be called to check on her son, who was in obvious distress the day before he died. More than that, Helen observed, "My clear impression was that the younger resident was afraid of disturbing the senior resident and the senior resident was afraid of disturbing the attending physician."

Health care professionals have much to learn from other industries in which it is expected that coworkers check on one another's work and intervene if a potential mistake is in progress, without fear that someone's ego will be hurt. It's an ingredient for disaster when doctors are reluctant to ask for help when they find themselves in over their heads. The "sink-or-swim" culture in medical training creates a climate of fear of seeking help, reluctance to question authority, and unwillingness to accept good advice even if it comes from someone of a different tribe or down a few notches in the hierarchy.

A veteran doctor reflects on the understandable fear and hesitancy among some residents to question senior doctors, saying, "I've seen situations where if a resident told the attending that something he did was not right, he or she could be kicked out of the residency program or severely reprimanded."

Dangerous Sleep Deprivation

Every spring Americans move their clocks forward one hour over a weekend in the annual ritual that accompanies the switch to daylight-saving time. The following Monday, there is an increase in motor vehicle accidents. This is no coincidence. Even minimal sleep deprivation affects performance. Too little sleep has been linked to public catastrophes. The Exxon Valdez oil spill, the nuclear accident at Chernobyl, and the close call at Three Mile Island have been associated with workers' sleep deficits.

Many industries recognize the impact of working too many hours without sleep. Airlines cannot schedule pilots to fly more than a certain number of hours in a week, month, and year. Train operators and other workers whose jobs affect public safety have limits on the maximum number of hours they can work.

Health care is different. Sleep deprivation is widespread among residents. After four years of medical school, residents spend anywhere from three to seven more years in training, usually in hospitals and other health care facilities. The 100,000 residents who are in training provide a significant amount of care around the clock in teaching hospitals. When residents were surveyed, 70 percent said they saw a colleague working in an impaired condition, and the cause of impairment reported most often was lack of sleep.[8]

Many young doctors in training say that sleep deprivation causes them to make mistakes. We call this "taking the red eye in the hospital." Late-night "red eye" flights can be a good way to fly to the East Coast from the West Coast. Most passengers usually sleep. They hope—and expect—that the pilots are more awake and alert than they themselves are.

There is no such prohibition in health care. Some doctors tend to patients when they have been awake far longer than the human mind and body can function effectively. One young resident described the effects of sleep deprivation this way, "I felt at times I was forced to give a level of medical care that was significantly less than I was capable of because I didn't have enough time. At times I was pushed so far I couldn't care anymore. At times, I wished (never helped) that patients would die so that I could sleep!!"[9] Another soon-to-be-resident admits, "My mother is mostly worried about whether I will fall asleep and stick myself with a needle; *I'm* afraid that I will kill someone."

Sleep deprivation can have an effect on the human body similar to being drunk. Researchers have found that when people were awake for more than seventeen hours, cognitive psychomotor performance was similar to that of someone with a blood alcohol level of 0.05 percent. After twenty-fours hours of being awake, performance was equivalent to a blood alcohol level of 0.10 percent, which is more than many states' legal driving limits.

Doctors who defend the status quo say that grueling training helps young physicians withstand fatigue and meet the unpredictable needs of patients. Health care is not shift work, in which doctors can punch out when the clock strikes a certain time. Patients' needs don't go by the clock. Long and complicated operations might take hours to perform, and surgical teams must remain alert for long periods.

Here's how one orthopedic surgery resident from California described the training regimen to the American Medical Student Association: "I was operating postcall after being up for over thirty-six hours and was holding retractors. I literally fell asleep standing up and nearly face-planted into the wound. My upper arm hit the side of the gurney, and I caught myself before I fell to the floor. I nearly put my face in the open wound, which would have contaminated the entire field and could have resulted in an infection for the patient."

Some proponents of the status quo say that there are no good studies that show that patients are injured because doctors are sleep deprived. Advocates for long hours assert that a patient is better off having a tired physician who knows the patient rather than a physician who is well rested but isn't familiar with the details of a patient's illness and care. No doubt a patient and family would value that continuity. Yet high-hazard industries operate on the reasonable assumption that fatigue and sleep deprivation compromise performance, and can be deadly. This suggests that the burden of proof is on those who wish to maintain the status quo.

Imagine for a moment that you need surgery, and two equally qualified surgeons are available to perform the operation. One surgeon has been awake continuously for thirty hours, having just completed several difficult surgeries. The other surgeon just came to work after a good night's sleep. Which surgeon would you want operating on you?

FLOUTING THE LAW

In 1989, New York State adopted regulations limiting the number of hours that medical residents could work to eighty, averaged over a four-week period. A resident could not be assigned more than twenty-four consecutive hours of work. Residents must be supervised by senior physicians, who are required to be on site twenty-four hours a day, seven days a week. These changes were aimed at protecting the public's safety and were generated by the outcry over the death in 1984 of Libby Zion, an eighteen-year-old who was admitted to a New York City hospital with a high fever. She died from an adverse reaction between two medications that should not be taken together. The investigation found that the young doctor taking care of her was in training, sleep-deprived, and overworked. Young doctors in the hospital routinely worked more than one hundred hours a week.

Ten years after New York instituted these regulations, and spent $240 million a year for eight years so hospitals could hire more staff to take the place of tired residents, an unannounced state inspection of twelve hospitals found that none was complying with the law. The state health department interviewed more than five hundred and sixty residents, checked more than five hundred patients' records, and talked to more than two hundred supervising physicians. Senior doctors were personally supervising all surgical procedures involving general anesthesia, but residents, particularly those in New York City, were working far more hours than allowed by law. Twenty percent of residents in New York City were working in excess of ninety-five hours a week. Thirty-eight percent of all residents worked more than twenty-four consecutive hours.

Young doctors have it especially hard in New York City, where 77 percent of surgery residents reported working more than ninety-five hours a week; in hospitals in upstate New York, it was 32 percent. "How is it possible for anyone to be functional working a ninety-five-hour week?" asked Bertrand Bell, Distinguished Professor of Medicine at the Jacobi Medical Center, in the Bronx. He told the *New York Times*, "A bus driver can't do it. A pilot cannot do it. So why should a neophyte doctor do it?"[10]

When a patient faces a life-threatening illness, serious conversations about medical treatments and their implications will likely be needed. An exhausted doctor is not in the best shape to intervene effectively with a patient and family. He or she may not have much energy to deal with other people's problems, especially profound issues of life and death, since sleep deprivation diminishes feelings of empathy. An internal medicine resident in Philadelphia described to the American Medical Student Association the impact sleep deprivation has: "I have witnessed the erosion of professional values and behavior of both myself and my colleagues when fatigue begins to set in. As a result, it becomes exceptionally difficult to put forth the same amount of thought and offer the same emotional support to patients after a long thirty-six-hour shift. The most disheartening feeling as a resident physician is when you feel that your own patients have become the enemy. I mean [they become] the one thing that stands between you and a few hours' sleep."

In November 1999, the European Parliament voted to limit, by 2003, the maximum workweek for junior physicians. Here in the United States, medical students and others have called for federal legislation to restrict the number of consecutive hours a young physician can work. Restricting work hours garnered interest in Congress when Congressman John Conyers, Jr., a Democrat from Michigan, and Senator Jon Corzine, a Democrat from New Jersey, introduced legislation in 2002 to restrict the number of hours residents can work to eighty per week and no more than twenty-four consecutive hours on duty. Meanwhile, supporters of work-hour limits filed a petition to the federal Occupational Safety and Health

Administration to request that working conditions for doctors in training be regulated by the federal government, just as other workers' hours are regulated. The petition requested a limit of an eighty-hour workweek, one day off a week, and shifts of no more than twenty-four hours.

These legislative and regulatory remedies being sought coincided with action by the medical profession to regulate work hours more stringently, a step that has staved off government intervention. OSHA declined the petition because the medical profession is implementing new standards beginning in July 2003 that restrict working hours and reinforce the requirement that young doctors in training be adequately supervised.

A WAKE-UP CALL AT YALE

The organization that accredits the training programs for resident physicians, the Accreditation Council for Graduate Medical Education (ACGME), monitors resident training in nearly 7,800 programs throughout the United States. In 2000, it cited 8 percent of training programs for violating their own work-hour limits. At that point, it had yet to withdraw accreditation status from a physician training program because of violations of work-hour limits.

In the spring of 2002, things changed. The ACGME withdrew the accreditation of the general surgery residency training program at Yale-New Haven Hospital, a teaching affiliate of the Yale University School of Medicine. Surgeons in training were working more than a hundred hours a week and were inadequately supervised. ACGME gave the teaching program until the summer of 2002 to make major improvements in working conditions and to reduce the number of hours residents work to eighty hours.

The loss of accreditation hit Yale-New Haven like a lightning bolt. It is unthinkable for such a prestigious institution to lose its ability to train future surgeons. Without a surgery training program, its ability to teach medical students and attract cream-of-the-crop surgeons would be wiped out. According to the ACGME, the Yale-New Haven training program has since been given provisional accreditation status.

In June 2002, the ACGME announced strict new limits on work hours for all 7,800 residency training programs in the country. Beginning in July 2003, residents may not work more than eighty hours a week, and senior physicians will be required to provide sufficient supervision to the young doctors in training.

Will the limits be enforced, or will training programs continue the same habits? The ACGME will conduct Internet surveys of residents to monitor compliance with the new limits, but some residents are skeptical about whether enforcement will be stringent enough to ensure that hospitals comply. The failure of many of New York's hospitals to comply with statewide limits is not a distant memory.

Residents say they need a confidential way to report incidents when the hospitals in which they work violate the ACGME standards. Residents feel they need to be protected from retribution, especially since some residency training programs can have as few as ten to fifteen people. They recommend that reports of noncompliance be made public on a regular basis, because a sleep-deprived work force is a matter of public health. By regularly publicizing this information, the safety of residency training can remain in the public eye.

These changes are coming too late for a man who had surgery in January 2002 at a hospital in New York to donate part of his liver to his brother. Three days after the surgery, he choked on vomit and died. His brother lived. An inexperienced, first-year resident was the only physician present to care for thirty-four patients in serious condition. Senior doctors at the hospital did not adequately supervise the resident—a deficiency in the Yale-New Haven resident training program as well. Officials in the New York State Department of Health cited the hospital for woefully inadequate postsurgical care, and specifically, for leaving the care of its transplant patients to one "inadequately supervised and overbur-dened resident." This deficiency was compounded by a shortage of nurses on the unit. The ACGME requires training programs to provide "appropriate backup support when patient care responsi-bilities are especially difficult and prolonged."

Will other patients in the future bear the consequences of inad-equately supervised doctors in training? The profession has a poor track record in enforcing its own rules. On the other hand, highly publicized cases of unsupervised residents causing harm to patients, coupled with growing public demand for patient safety, has put res-idency training programs in the hot seat. They will remain there as long as the public is vigilant and its common-sense views continue to shape the norms that govern the training of future doctors in America.

6 | "A Nurse Saved My Life"

Terry is a Yale graduate and served as a navigator in World War II with a Naval air transport squadron based in Honolulu. The C-54 planes he navigated across the Pacific brought wounded soldiers home from Okinawa. Now seventy-eight years old and still working almost full-time, he remembers when he was admitted to a New Jersey hospital for quadruple heart bypass surgery eighteen years ago. The night after the surgery, Terry was in the cardiac unit. He recalls that in those days, hospitals didn't have monitors with loud alarms signaling cardiac arrest. In the middle of the night his heart stopped. Looking back on those life-and-death moments, Terry quietly says, "A nurse saved my life. She was keeping a close eye on me and saw that I was in distress. She called the code and they resuscitated me." A day later, when he was still groggy, Terry remembers the nurse saying to him, "Do you remember me? You were in pretty serious trouble." Terry had been in cardiac arrest for some time and the doctors were concerned he would have brain damage, if he survived at all. "She caught me in time," he says. "This is why I have such a high regard for the nursing profession. If I were in the hospital today with nurses overworked, I don't know if I would be so fortunate."

Sounding the Alarm

Nurses save lives such as Terry's and countless others every day. When too few nurses are available to take care of patients, their needs are overlooked, and medical mistakes occur. This is based not just on anecdote but on well-documented research.

Once again, a study published in a prestigious medical journal sounds the alarm. In October 2002, the *Journal of the American Medical Association* published the results of a study that for the first time showed that the number of patients who die in the hospital increases when nurses are assigned to care for too many patients.[1] An estimated 20,000 people die each year in hospitals from medical mistakes attributed to nurses caring for more patients than they can handle. This accounts for 20 percent of the nearly 100,000 deaths annually from medical mistakes. While a link between nurse staffing and the quality of care seems like common sense, many hospitals downplayed the link—until this study was published.

The researchers who conducted the study reviewed the medical records of more than 230,000 patients who were admitted into hospitals in Pennsylvania for routine procedures such as knee replacement and gall bladder removal. They found that when nurses were taking care of eight patients, there was a 31 percent greater risk of patients dying than when nurses were overseeing the care of just four patients.

These findings reveal the importance of having enough nurses with sufficient time to closely monitor patients. They also show that many mistakes are not simply the result of incompetent or careless individuals, but result instead from the failure of health care organizations to be adequately staffed to provide quality care.

An earlier *Chicago Tribune* report in September 2000 examined the impact of the nursing shortage. To help monitor patients' vital signs, hospitals have machines such as blood-oxygen monitors. Even with advances in technology and monitoring devices—some of which didn't exist when Terry, the WWII aviation navigator, was

hospitalized—nurses' ability to monitor patient care doesn't necessarily improve if too few nurses are taking care of too many
patients. Scores of patients around the country have died or been
injured when nurses haven't heard the warning alarms that are
built into the lifesaving machines. One example reported by the
Tribune is a patient who died of a heart attack after the alarm on a
respiratory machine sounded. The only nurse on duty was responsible for caring for ten patients, and she told investigators that she
was tending to another patient in distress at the time and didn't
hear the other patient's alarm.

In Florida, Clara, an active ninety-four-year-old great-grand-
mother who still worked as a hospital volunteer two days a week,
was admitted to the hospital for a bowel obstruction. She and her
family, along with nurses from the hospital, said that there were too
few nurses to check her during the night when her eldest son went
home to sleep for a couple of hours. Clara called the nurses to help
her use the bathroom but when no one came, she climbed over the
bed railing. Still groggy from surgery twenty hours earlier, Clara fell
to the floor and broke her left hip. She died two days later during
surgery to repair the hip fracture. "It was just too much for her,"
said her grandson. "For want of one nurse, she died."

Not all consequences of the nursing shortage are life-threatening. Sometimes the impact of the shortage is demeaning to the
dignity of patients and their families. In some intensive care units,
nurses tie patients' arms and legs to the bed so they don't move
too much and displace intravenous tubes and monitoring devices.
This is a consequence of too few nurses caring for too many
patients, and they can't be sufficiently vigilant for each and every
patient.

A former nurse described her experience with the shortage this
way: "I was visiting my mother while she was in the hospital in
New Jersey. I asked the floor nurse if she could help me put my
mother on the commode. She was so overworked and said that
they were not staffed to put patients on the commode and that my

mother should 'go in her bed and we'll clean it up later.' I was trained as a nurse years ago and can't believe what has happened to nursing care."

Here's what a nurse said about why patients' needs are not met. "Just imagine there are two nurses and a couple of aides to take care of thirty very ill patients, four of whom are on a ventilator. It's not possible to do everything that needs to be done."

Family members pick up the slack. Ockie's family, whom you met in Chapter 2, moved him to a health care facility where, as his daughter, Rebecca, says, "They just had too many patients per caregiver to take care of anyone. It was so sad. Some days were better than others. I don't know if it was scheduling problems, not enough nurses, or too many nurses calling in sick. We remember clearly how important it was to have Dad turned from side to side to prevent bed sores, but we would spend hours up there and no one would come in to do it."

Turning Away Patients

The U.S. health care system is facing an unprecedented shortage of nurses especially in hospitals, and the American Hospital Association estimates that there are 126,000 vacant positions for registered nurses, which is a vacancy rate of about 11 percent. The shortage is so severe in some parts of the country that hospitals have had to turn away patients because they don't have enough nurses to care for them. The Johns Hopkins Hospital in Baltimore, a hospital top-ranked by *U.S. News and World Report*, is one of them. It had brand-new, high-tech hospital rooms in its surgical intensive care unit. But the doors to this unit were shut for a period of time because the hospital couldn't hire enough nurses to take care of the patients.

The situation at Johns Hopkins Hospital is not uncommon. California's hospitals have about a 20 percent nursing staff vacancy rate, and many hospitals in New York don't have enough nurses to staff emergency departments, operating rooms, and intensive care units. Even the $10,000 signing bonuses being offered by some hospitals are not enough to attract a sufficient number of nurses. They create an incentive for nurses to go from one hospital to the next—hardly a strategy to instill long-term loyalty.

If you ask hospital administrators if there is a shortage of nurses in their facilities, they may tell you that the hospital is operating within the "industry norm." This means that the hospital is in the same predicament as most other hospitals nationally, which are feeling the pinch of a serious shortage of nurses. Based on the study mentioned earlier, it's safe to say that that "norm" is killing people. This is not much comfort to someone in the hospital who is suffering from inadequate care nor to someone who has been the victim of a medical mistake because of a lack of nurses.

We spoke with a well-informed nurse who knows the inside workings of many hospitals in a major urban area on the East Coast. We asked if she recommends that people anticipating a hospital stay arrange for a private-duty nurse to be with them, especially after surgery. "*Absolutely*," she says. "People don't want to hear how bad it is, but it's true. My brother had surgery recently at a hospital that has a good reputation and we were there all the time just to be sure."

Why Are Nurses Leaving the Bedside?

Experienced nurses as well as newly minted nurses are leaving patient care at the bedside at a time when other job opportunities exist. Their knowledge and skills are valued in pharmaceutical companies, managed care organizations, and information technology firms. How many are leaving? It is hard to say precisely. The federal government's Bureau of Health Professions issued a report showing that about 50,000 fewer nurses were using their licenses in 2000 as compared with 1996.

AT THE MERCY OF MANAGEMENT

Many hospitals have conditions that are ripe for medical mistakes to occur, and these conditions are driving nurses out of hospital care because they can't always provide the quality care they were trained to give. Nurses want to do good—to save people's lives, just as the nurse who saved Terry's life did. The last thing good nurses want to do is jeopardize the health of their patients. But this is exactly what can—and does—happen. As one nurse said, "Nurses didn't go into the profession to be witnesses to suffering from the care being provided."

In a Denver hospital, a newborn infant died as a result of a medication error. Three nurses who were taking care of the infant were indicted for criminally negligent homicide. Two of the nurses accepted a guilty plea, the terms of which included a two-year probationary period, because they didn't want the third nurse, who had a negligible role in the error, to be found guilty by association. Experts on medical errors who were helping the nurse who stood trial conducted an in-depth analysis of the cause of the mistake and uncovered fifty separate failures in the hospital that contributed to the error.[2] If any one of these failures had been detected, the infant would not have suffered harm. Some of the failures included a drug order—handwritten by a physician—that was unclear, a pharmacist who filled the order with a tenfold overdose, and the absence of a warning system to alert the pharmacist to the overdose.

After hearing this analysis, and after only forty-five minutes of deliberations, the jury found the nurse on trial not guilty. More than that, the jurors demonstrated their personal support for the nurse by tearfully hugging her after they rendered their verdict. They recognized that the nurse was not to blame, because she was working in an organization whose management did not put systems in place that could have prevented the chain of mistakes that led to the tragic error.

STRETCHED TOO THIN

Operating within the industry norm does little to reassure nurses who are responsible for patient care. For one twenty-year nursing veteran, the stress of providing care while short-staffed drove her to a more sedate job in a doctor's office. Another nurse exclaims, "How I loved being a nurse! But I would never practice as a nurse in certain parts of the country. I know hospitals where the care is atrocious. Nurses are having to do everything—take care of thirteen med-surg patients while at the same time answer the phones, take a patient down to X-ray because no one else shows up to do it, handle emergencies, talk to families, administer medications, make sure the medications on the unit are not expired...you name it."

These nurses are not alone in feeling the stresses of the job, which was another finding from the study on the impact of nurse staffing on patients' safety. When a hospital increases a nurse's workload by just one patient, this increases the chances that the nurse is dissatisfied by 15 percent, and the odds of burnout by 23 percent. When nurses working in Pennsylvania were surveyed for another study, 22 percent of the 14,000 nurses who responded said they were planning to quit within the next year. Nationally, the American Nurses Association found that 71 percent of nurses said they felt "exhausted, discouraged, or powerless to change their working conditions."

The California legislature has realized the negative consequences for patients when nurses have too many patients to care for. It is the first state to pass a law that requires hospitals to abide by a maximum number of patients per nurse. Exactly what the ratio should be is being debated, and the study findings about how the risk to patients varies depending upon the nurse-to-patient ratio may offer useful insight in this debate.

Cutting to the Bone

Labor costs account for more than half the cost of operating a hospital. Not surprisingly, then, when hospitals have to cut costs, the first thing they scrutinize is staffing numbers. Managed care organizations have put hospitals in a financial vise in recent years. On another front, hospitals face cuts in the growth in Medicare funding to care for the elderly.

Registered nurses constitute a substantial percentage of hospital employees and are the single biggest labor cost to the hospital. With increased responsibility for more seriously ill patients, and fewer supporting staff, hospital nurses are struggling. It comes as no surprise that the level of trust between nurses and hospital management has eroded in many institutions.

FORCED OVERTIME

As hospitals have cut back on nurses, the remaining nurses bear a larger burden, and a vicious cycle ensues. The overworked staff leave and the nurses left behind have an even larger burden. This burden has taken the form of more hospitals imposing mandatory overtime on the remaining nurses. While nurses might voluntarily work overtime, they are increasingly forced to work overtime. If they don't, the hospitals would have to stop admitting patients. A veteran nurse said, "Imagine what it is like when you're suddenly at the end of your shift and you are told you have to work another eight hours, and meanwhile, your eight-year-old little boy is waiting for you at home. If you say no, then you are threatened with the loss of your nursing license because you are abandoning your patients. But the hospital put the schedule up a while ago and they knew then that they didn't have anyone to cover."

Mandatory overtime in hospitals is sometimes inevitable because the number of patients admitted to a hospital fluctuates and is unpredictable. While hospitals once had staff who were available to cover periodic increases in hospital admissions during the flu season, for example, now they typically maintain enough nursing staff only to cover core functions, if even that much. When patient admissions spike, the core staff have to cope. Mandatory overtime has become a way of solving a much bigger problem than it was intended to solve, and it is driving away the very nurses that are needed. As Congressman Tom Lantos of California has said, "At a time when hospitals are trying to reduce medical errors, forced overtime makes no sense."

Confessions of a Consultant

Many hospitals hire health care consultants to help them downsize or, to use politically correct language, "right-size" their organization. As with any consultants, if they don't thoroughly understand what it takes to give patients good care, their recommendations can be detrimental. A nationally recognized leader in the nursing profession, Claire Fagin, recounted this story in a report she wrote for the Milbank Memorial Fund in 2001:

"I once had a chance conversation with a man who, I learned, had in the past worked for one of the major consulting companies and had been deeply involved in the restructuring of a number of hospitals. Learning that I was a nurse, he said, somewhat sheepishly, 'I'm one of the bad guys.' He told me about what he described as 'his naive and dangerous' period and was filled with guilt over the restructuring recommendations he had made in his former job. His awakening, he said, had come when his wife had had a baby who required intensive, long-term neonatal care. During the hours and days the couple spent at the hospital with their critically vulnerable infant, they had a chance to see nurses at work expertly caring for—and ultimately saving—their child's life. In the process, he came to understand what nurses do and how important their job is."

Skewed Priorities

In the feverishness of cutting costs, hospital administrators who don't have the same understanding as this consultant say that they often cut staff rather than funding for capital improvements or research. The core work of hospitals—patient care—is getting short shrift. Certainly health care facilities need capital improvements. Some hospitals are designing more patient-friendly facilities. And who can argue against more research? But if it comes at the expense of the core purpose of health care—patient care—is that the right allocation of resources? There is hardly anything more patient-friendly than having knowledgeable health care professionals with the time to properly care for a sick patient.

Why does this misallocation of resources occur? Hospitals want to attract patients and doctors so they build state-of-the-art facilities. They compete for more research dollars and prestigious medical researchers. But they don't compete on the basis of the quality of care provided to patients. If they did, they wouldn't be cutting back on patient care. And patients wouldn't be dying or being injured at the rate they are now because of medical mistakes. It's not that we don't spend enough money on health care. The priorities aren't right.

A local hospital outside Washington, D.C., mailed a nice glossy brochure to nearby residents. It described the hospital's plan to spend $150 million for a new facility. All rooms will be private, a 1,100-car parking garage will be attached to the hospital so visitors and patients won't have to walk in the rain, and the hospital will be equipped with state-of-the-art technology. The brochure features an architect's drawing of the atrium and breezeway to show that the facility will be aesthetically pleasing.

ork
ate-

the
that
ality
lized
fairs,
con-
ospi-
are a
ours.
with
ant. I
y ori-
nurse
ndle a
lomen
about
"Okay,
fusely,

wards,
njuries
surgery
n grew
regard-
ft, who
for the
er man-
tically.
y others
d to the
uld sur-

spital's nurse vacancy and turnover rate?
es has been required to work mandatory
months? What is the hospital's infection
sting in computer technology proven to
s? If the public were asked how they
nditures to be spent, it's not hard to guess
th care can mean the difference between
its and families want to know whether
re possible. Certainly that's more mean-
t.

y

how the nursing shortage is affecting
he shortage is having a big impact, but
ses in his hospital were leaving. Imag-
aid the same thing about flight atten-
ir jobs in droves. When an exodus of
that a systemic human resource prob-
atter of a few disgruntled employees.
problem, planes would be grounded
undles of money. You can bet the air-
ottom of why an essential part of his
ng and make amends. But that doesn't
it's not just budget cuts that are dri-
ospital leadership is clueless about the
of its most precious resources.
e and the respect it has for its work-
rale. The work that nurses do can be
nd that, in itself, is cause to render
keep good nurses and attract new
nslated into meaningful roles and
in decision making about patient

care, increased autonomy, and more predictable and flexi
schedules. Wise health care administrators are using the
gies successfully to attract and retain good nurses.

The mismatch between patients' needs and the ski
nurses taking care of them is a telltale sign of an organiza
is in trouble. When the "father" of the movement to brir
assurance to health care, Dr. Avedis Donabedian, was ho
and interviewed in a leading health policy journal, *Heal*
he was asked the following question: "What was your ser
fidence in the day-to-day management of your care in t
tal?" His response was telling. "I think the hospital flo
disaster. I saw so many part-time nurses working variab
They come and go. Often I couldn't tell whether I was de
a nurse, a technician, an attending physician, or an att
saw rampant discontinuity in nursing care and many p
ented nurses, especially on weekends. I had a you
assigned to me one day who clearly did not know how to
colostomy [which is surgery to create an opening in the
to allow for waste elimination]. "Do you know anyth
colostomy management?" I asked her. "No," she answer
sit down. I'll teach you." She learned and thanked me
but this was an unbelievable situation."

In some hospitals, nurses are rotated between differe
depending on staffing requirements. A woman whos
required a twelve-day hospital stay following complicat
had a new nurse each shift for nine days, until her sur
tired of the poor care his patient was receiving, particula
ing her pain medication. The head nurse of each s
remained constant from day to day, assumed responsibi
care of this patient and, not surprisingly, her pain was b
aged and her spirits and rate of recovery improved dran

It would be hard to argue that this situation, and m
like it, was the fault of the nurses who were newly assig
orthopedic ward each day. Hardly any other business v

vive if its workers were so mismatched with its customers' needs. Just imagine a homeowner who calls a plumber to fix a leak, and the person who comes is a heating-and-air-conditioning expert who knows nothing about plumbing. The homeowner certainly wouldn't pay for the house call and probably wouldn't patronize that business again. But, no doubt, in the example of mismatched nursing care, the patient's insurance reimbursed the hospital for the cost of the hospital care, including the ill-prepared staff. Where else would this happen besides in health care?

Would You Coach a Football Team This Way?

Instead of trying to preserve its precious assets, hospitals often hire temporary nurses, which can add fuel to the fire of mismatches between patients' needs and the skills of nurses caring for them. The demand for temporary nurses has skyrocketed to unprecedented levels, and temp agencies can't keep up with the demand and can fill only a small fraction of the requests they receive. Hospitals pay top dollar for these services, and the high pay scale and benefits for temporary nurses can cause resentment among permanent nursing staff.

Temporary nurses can be an appropriate remedy in states like Arizona and Florida when people from colder northern climates migrate to warmer climates to escape the ice and snow in the winter months. But relying on temporary nurses to remedy a nursing shortage is about as effective as driving a car with one of those small spare tires. It won't take anyone very far.

Since health care is becoming more businesslike, it seems reasonable that good business practices would be adopted. Hospitals are using the staffing models of other industries by cutting fixed labor costs to save money. Temporary outsourced workers do work that fluctuates. But the application of the business model to health care doesn't work so well. Patients are not widgets on an assembly line. Continuity of care by the same health care professional is essential for effective monitoring of patients during their recovery.

Imagine a football coach trying to find replacements for missing team members right before a big game. Imagine the coach having to do this every week. A team like this wouldn't win very often and would probably make a lot more mistakes than a seasoned team that practiced and played together. Many hospitals have to work with such a "last-minute team" as administrators struggle every day to find enough registered nurses to fill the record-breaking vacancies.

Many Americans probably have had firsthand experience with the nursing shortage but may not have realized it. If you or someone you know has checked into a hospital recently, you may have noticed that hospitals are relying on larger numbers of lower-cost, unlicensed staff instead of registered nurses. A patient care technician or unlicensed aide might check on a patient rather than a registered nurse. The care that unlicensed staff provide to patients can be very valuable, but if they are put in a position of rendering care for which they are not adequately trained, patients can be harmed and a disservice is done to the caregiver.

Robbing Peter to Pay Paul

When faced with a shortage of workers, America, the land of immigrants, looks overseas for recruits. During the technology boom, Congress allowed skilled computer programmers and technicians from overseas to enter the United States to fill vacant jobs. Farmers need workers to harvest crops, so Congress gives the nod to programs that allow migrant workers to help put food on America's kitchen tables.

While there is no shortage of high-tech or agricultural workers worldwide, there is a worldwide shortage of nurses. Some poor countries are witnessing a "brain drain" of nurses, as recruiters from the United States and Europe scour hospitals in countries as far away as the Philippines, Ghana, and South Africa. The cost to poor countries is high. Already burdened by too few nurses, and with limited funds to build new nursing schools, poor countries are losing some of their best and brightest nurses. The *Wall Street Journal* reported in January 2001 that countries such as Trinidad have seen half of their nurses leave for other countries. In countries where earnings are low and working conditions less than ideal, many nurses leap at the chance to work in the United States.

The number of nurses who have left Ghana to take more lucrative jobs in Europe and the United States was more than twice the number of graduates from Ghana's nursing schools that same year. Some hospitals in Ghana have had to close entire hospital floors because there aren't enough nurses. Nurses from Ghana go to Britain; British nurses go to Canada; and Canadian nurses come to the United States. The bottom line is that overseas recruitment is a stopgap measure for hospitals and won't solve the nursing shortage here at home. It's also worth noting here that the education and training programs overseas may not provide nursing students with the knowledge and skills they may need to care for patients in this country.

What Price Value?

As hospitals try to respond to the nursing shortage, it's like locking the barn door after the horses have bolted. Not only are the horses gone, but they may never come back. One well-regarded physician, who served as dean of a medical school on the West Coast, was diagnosed with cancer and underwent a painful ordeal of surgery and chemotherapy. One of his junior colleagues asked him what he had learned from that experience. He replied that the most important thing was, "Respect the nurses." Not known as a physician willing to work collaboratively with nurses, he finally realized firsthand the value of nursing. A face-to-face encounter with death is a great equalizer.

Ask David Letterman. When he returned to late-night television after his heart bypass surgery, he invited the doctors and nurses who cared for him onto his show, introduced them to his audience, and hugged his bedside nurse.

If you talk to seasoned nurses, perhaps those who have retired or who have left patient care, you notice wistfulness, even sadness, for the old days of real nursing. Many nurses remember how they once could care for patients in the way they were trained. They are saddened by the loss of something intangible that nurses brought to caring for patients. Nurses have always been a huge part of the "care" in health care, and they still are. The health care industry has cut back on the care that nurses were once allowed to give their patients because there is no direct monetary value in such services. Yet, no one can put a price on caring or translate it into dollars and cents.

The health care system cannot shoulder the entire blame for this dilemma. Health care is a reflection of society and its values. Our society puts less value on professions that teach, care, and nurture. It is no surprise that these occupations have traditionally been filled by women. Money matters in American culture, and it defines one's worth. Indeed, for many health care executives, the value of health care professionals today depends on whether they are a source of revenue or an expense. If they generate revenue, they are more valuable to a health care organization. The more revenue they generate, the more prestige is bestowed upon them. Physicians are more valued than nurses, in part because they are a source of revenue. They bring in patients who are paying customers. Nurses are not a revenue source. They are considered an expense and are listed on the other side of the balance sheet. Hospitals have to live with financial realities to survive. But is this good for patient care? Is this how the public would define value?

The different value placed on nurses is evident when medical mistakes are made. Nurses say that they bear more consequences than their physician counterparts when a mistake is made. "Things roll downhill, and nurses are the scapegoats," one nurse confided. "That's just the way it is."

The Next Generation

While nurses are leaving care at the bedside, there is yet another reason for the nursing shortage: fewer people are entering the profession. Looking ahead, if we think the nursing shortage is bad now, we haven't seen anything yet. It will become much more serious when older nurses retire, just as the baby boomers really show signs of aging.

The number of students enrolling in four-year nursing schools has been declining 5 percent a year since 1995, although an increase of almost 4 percent in 2001 from the prior year has offered a spark of hope—but it's too early to tell if this is just a short-term upward blip. Meanwhile, nursing schools don't have enough faculty. In fact, in the 2000–2001 academic year, nursing schools turned away about 6,000 applicants because there weren't enough faculty. And since the current generation of nursing faculty is retiring, and would-be nurse educators are shying away from teaching jobs, the situation is only going to get worse. Nursing schools can't offer faculty salaries that are competitive with the salaries offered to nurses who are directly caring for patients.

Women traditionally have filled the role of nurses, and today they constitute about 95 percent of registered nurses. Yet women today have many more career options than their counterparts twenty years ago. Those who would have been nurses twenty years ago are becoming doctors today. Women now account for 48 percent of first-year medical students, compared with 28 percent in 1980.

The critical shortage of nurses now is a harbinger of things to come. With fewer young people entering the nursing profession, the average age of registered nurses is forty-five years and is increasing. Just ask any nurse. Age matters. As one nurse admitted,

"I could work twelve-hour shifts with no problem when I was in my twenties. But now, almost twenty years later, I would be flat-out exhausted if I had to take care of so many patients."

In about ten years, the largest age group of nurses will be in their fifties and sixties and will begin to retire. Not enough nurses are being trained today to fill in the gaps and take care of tomorrow's aging baby boomers. In just fifteen years, many baby boomers will reach age sixty-five, become eligible for Medicare, and become susceptible to all the diseases and frailties that come with aging. The nursing shortage is not just a problem for the nursing profession or hospitals. It is everyone's problem.

Nurses are lobbying Congress to obtain some relief, and in December 2001, Congress passed the Nurse Reinvestment Act, which was designed to give scholarships to nurses who work in areas where there is an acute shortage, provide funding to recruit more nurses, and support more training for nurses. President Bush signed the Act into law in August 2002, but it wasn't until February 2003 that Congress appropriated money to fund some of the programs authorized in the Act.

Legislation can help resolve some of the reasons for the nursing shortage. But it won't solve a problem caused by inadequate people management in health care facilities. Nurses are saying they just can't take care of patients properly. And they want someone to listen.

Some enlightened leaders and managers of health care organizations are listening. A hospital in New Jersey reports that it has a waiting list of nurses who want to work in some of its units. What do they do differently? The CEO of the hospital understood years ago that if you want a good hospital you have to realize that, "It's about the nurses." And he's right.

7 | Death by Decimal

Medication errors are one of the most common medical mistakes, and they occur when drugs are prescribed, dispensed, and administered. When used correctly, prescription medications can mean the difference between life and death; when used incorrectly, they can mean the difference between life and death.

A nine-month-old girl died at a hospital in Washington, D.C., because a 0.5 milligram dose of morphine was mistakenly read as 5 milligrams. According to the *Washington Post*, a surgeon ordered 0.5 milligrams of morphine. This was the correct dosage, but it was written without a zero preceding the decimal point. A unit clerk transcribed the order at 5 milligrams. The nurse followed the order and gave 5 milligrams of morphine. When an overdose of morphine is given, it slows the respiratory system until it stops working and the patient can die from a lack of oxygen.

In cases such as this, the medication mistake is referred to as "death by decimal," and is one of many different types of error that can occur in the seemingly simple process of giving a patient a prescription drug. Yet, in reality, it is teeming with possibilities for error. Errors range from an illegible handwritten prescription, doctors' lack of knowledge about the appropriate use of a drug, confusion over different drugs with very similar names, pharmacist error in filling the prescription, and patients misusing medications because they are not taught how to use them correctly.

Given our national hunger for the latest elixir, it shouldn't be surprising that medication mistakes are not uncommon. Retail pharmacies—the corner drug store, chain drug stores in the shopping mall, and pharmacies in supermarkets—dispense nearly three billion prescriptions a year. This is in addition to the more than four billion doses of medications administered in hospitals. This huge volume coincides with the growth in the number of different prescription drugs that are available—almost a 500 percent increase in the last ten years. Now there are about 17,000 trade and generic names for prescriptions drugs, according to the Institute for Safe Medication Practices, a Pennsylvania-based nonprofit group that analyzes medication errors and recommends strategies to doctors, nurses, pharmacists, and others on how they can prevent them.

More diseases and conditions than ever are treated from the nation's prescription drug medicine cabinet. With more prescription drugs being prescribed by doctors, dispensed by pharmacists and administered by nurses or patients and their family members, more opportunities exist for serious medication mistakes to occur. Meanwhile, a shortage of qualified pharmacists is increasing the risk of mistakes in drug dispensing.

In its report, the IOM estimated that 7,000 people die in hospitals and elsewhere from medication mistakes. As with the other estimates, this is quite likely an undercount of the true number of mistakes for the same reasons that other medical errors are underestimated.

Inappropriate Prescribing

Many medication mistakes are made because doctors can't possibly remember all the names and purposes of drugs available, their side effects, and interactions with other drugs and over-the-counter medications. But this is the context in which prescription drugs are prescribed every day all across America. As we were writing this book, a neighbor mentioned that his wife, who has asthma, was prescribed a medication that should *never* be prescribed to someone with asthma. The couple switched physicians in the hope of finding one who is more careful. They are like many other older Americans who are prescribed drugs inappropriately. A study published in the *Journal of the American Medical Association* reported that almost 25 percent of older Americans not living in nursing homes or other institutional settings are prescribed potentially inappropriate drugs.

To understand why drugs are prescribed inappropriately, the American Society of Health-System Pharmacists conducted a survey, which found that 34 percent of seniors are taking medications prescribed by two or more physicians. When prescription and nonprescription medications are counted, along with dietary supplements, 76 percent of older adults take at least three medications, and about 33 percent take eight or more. Chances are very high that their doctors don't know that they're taking medications prescribed by other doctors.

Even if a doctor has access to a patient's medical record with the medication history, patients are still being prescribed drugs inappropriately. In one study of patients who went to the emergency department and were given medications, 10 percent were prescribed a new drug that could have had a negative interaction with a medication they were already taking.[1]

In Chapter 4 you met Marlene, who died in the hospital, about to give birth to her third child. Her family's story doesn't end there, as the family had a close brush with near-tragedy after her death. Her son was not feeling well, and her husband, Leonard, now bearing the sole responsibility for their three children, brought him to the hospital outpatient clinic. The boy was examined and given a prescription for a medication to help him feel better. When Leonard took the prescription to be filled at the hospital pharmacy, the pharmacist exclaimed, "This is enough for a horse!" The pharmacist called the doctor and the dosage error was corrected. This is a common error made when drugs are prescribed. For Leonard, it was unbelievable that the system failed him yet again.

Many medication errors are the result of mistakes in communicating and transcribing accurate information about the name of the drug and the dose. A tragic and highly publicized medication error occurred in November 1994 at the Dana-Farber Cancer Institute in Boston, which is affiliated with Harvard Medical School. Betsy Lehman was a seasoned health columnist for the *Boston Globe* and the thirty-nine-year-old mother of two. She underwent experimental chemotherapy treatment for breast cancer. Three weeks later she died, not from the cancer, but from a lethal overdose of an anticancer drug that was ordered and administered incorrectly by the staff.

This medication mistake occurred when the doctor wrote down the dose of chemotherapy that was to be given to the patient over the four-day period of therapy. However, the prescription was written on a form used to prescribe daily dosages, and as a result, the patient was given four times the prescribed amount of a highly toxic anticancer drug. She also received an incorrect dose of another drug that was administered to reduce the adverse effects of the chemotherapy. Another patient undergoing the same treatment also received the same wrong dose of chemotherapy. This patient survived but was greatly debilitated and subsequently died in 1997. Even with built-in checks in the system, where pharmacists and nurses check and recheck drug dosages, no one noticed the mistake.

The medication error that caused the patient's death was not discovered until three months later, when data on the patient was entered into a computer at Dana-Farber. The error in dosage was identified. The cause of death was cardiac toxicity resulting from the overdose.

Dana-Farber used this tragic mistake as a wake-up call and has since overhauled its system to prevent such errors from happening again. The organization's board, leadership, and staff reviewed policies and procedures, and instituted top-to-bottom improvements to prevent tragic errors.

The Massachusetts legislature enacted a law in December 2001 establishing the Betsy Lehman Center for Patient Safety and Medical Error Reduction, so named in honor of the *Boston Globe* reporter. Its role will be to coordinate statewide efforts to increase awareness among health care professionals and the public of strategies to prevent errors. With states such as Massachusetts facing a serious fiscal crisis, coupled with the absence so far of a strong political constituency to lobby for initiatives to prevent medical mistakes, the legislature has yet to appropriate any money to fund the center.

Cleaning Up the Chicken Scratch

Imagine if the U.S. banking and brokerage industry still relied on handwriting to record transactions. What if customers received handwritten checking account statements every month? Think of how many mistakes would be made: a decimal point in the wrong place, a "1" mistaken for a "7," numbers transposed. Imagine a retired couple receiving a handwritten retirement account statement and instead of showing the $250,000 they had saved over a lifetime, it showed a balance of $25,000. Chances are the error would be fixed by a telephone call, but not until the couple's hearts skipped a few beats.

Mistakes are also made with drugs that end in the letter "l," when pharmacists mistake the "l" for the numeral "1." In two recent cases reported by the Institute for Safe Medication Practices, pharmacists mistakenly filled a prescription for the antiseizure drug *Tegretol 300 milligrams* with *1300 milligrams*, and the diabetes drug *Amaryl 2 milligrams* with *12 milligrams*. Patients suffered from drug overdoses in both cases.

When prescriptions for medications are handwritten, errors occur with frightening frequency. Each year, pharmacists make an estimated 150 million phone calls to doctors because they can't read their handwriting, according to the Institute for Safe Medication Practices. If the doctor and pharmacist each spend one minute on each call, and if 150 million phone calls are made each year to decipher doctors' hieroglyphics, this is the equivalent of one person spending 570 years on the phone, at an enormous cost and loss of productivity.

Illegible scrawl might be a badge of prestige for some doctors who are overworked and always in a rush. But it is an expensive and sometimes deadly form of prestige. To drive home this point, the physician chief of staff at a California hospital held a contest. He offered a free lunch at an upscale restaurant for anyone on his staff who could decipher medical instructions written by doctors with the most illegible handwriting. No one could read them. The hospital started a course on good handwriting.

Other hospitals are also seeing the handwriting on the wall. A Connecticut hospital hosted handwriting seminars taught by an expert on penmanship. In these three-hour seminars, doctors and physician assistants learned the art of writing clear script. One hopes the prescriptions the doctors write and the orders they put in patients' medical records will now be easily read.

But penmanship courses are a stopgap measure, not a solution, and, in fact, can give a false sense of security to the hospital, believing that it has solved the problem of bad handwriting.

To eliminate these medication errors, especially mistakes from illegible chicken scratch, all prescription ordering in hospitals should be computerized. It's hard to believe that although 4 billion individual doses of medication are administered in hospitals every year, only 2 percent to 5 percent of hospitals have computerized prescription-ordering systems. The American Pharmaceutical Association, the professional society of pharmacists, has proposed an end to handwritten prescriptions nationwide by 2005. It's unlikely that this goal will be met, but it's the right goal to achieve.

Patients with the Same Name

Despite some of the high-tech computer systems they use, some hospitals seem unable to prevent doctors from prescribing the wrong medication to patients in the hospital who have the same name. One doctor described the following case.

"One weekend, I saw a patient who had a relatively unusual name. The patient had pain, anxiety, and agitation, and I recommended changes to her medications. I spoke to the intern and resident caring for her on Saturday and they promised to take care of the change in the orders. On Sunday morning I saw the patient and she did not seem better. I logged onto the computer under the patient's name on Sunday to see if the meds had been changed. None of the ones I had recommended had been ordered. I was upset and went ahead and put the orders into the computer even though that is normally the job of the interns and the residents. After I did that I paged the resident to ask what had happened. She said, 'We did put the orders in. I think you are looking at the wrong patient.' I checked the computer again, and she was right. There were two patients with the same relatively unusual name in the hospital and I had entered the orders for powerful drugs for the wrong patient. Fortunately, I was able to cancel them in time. The computer did not warn me that there were two patients with the identical name in the hospital. I was supposed to remember to look and notice that myself. This error could have caused great harm and was caught only by luck and serendipity. When I pushed for a systems response—routine notification to prescribing physicians when there is more than one patient by the same name in the hospital at the same time—I was told that the system memory required to run all names against the total list each time any prescriber logged on would slow the system down to unusable speeds."

And that's where the matter rests in one of the nation's leading teaching hospitals.

Drugs with Similar Names

Just as patients' names can be mistaken for each other, so can similar-sounding names of prescription drugs. When a pharmacist or nurse can't read a doctor's handwriting, the task of deciphering the name of a drug that is similar to another very different drug can be difficult. The difference between *amoxicillin* and *ampicillin*, for example, is not that much when handwriting is illegible. A cardiologist had to pay $225,000 to the family of a patient who died after receiving *Plendil*, a medication for high blood pressure, instead of *Isordil*, which is used to prevent or treat chest pain, because the pharmacist misinterpreted the doctor's handwriting.

Confusion over the names of similar-sounding drugs is a very common cause of drug-related mistakes. The sound-alike names for *Lamictal*, a drug used to treat epilepsy, and *Lamisil*, used to treat fungal infections, are a case in point. The volume of dispensing errors involving these two drugs prompted warnings to pharmacists of the potential confusion.

Another medication mistake, reported to U.S. Pharmacopeia (a nongovernmental group based in Rockville, Maryland, which maintains a medication error-reporting program), occurred when an order for *amiodarone* was called into a hospital pharmacy for a patient in distress in the emergency department. The pharmacist mistakenly dispensed *amrinone*, then realized the error and got to the emergency department before the patient was given the drug. After a number of similar mix-ups across the country with these two drugs, which are used to treat different cardiac problems, the name of the drug *amrinone* was changed to *inamrinone*.

Medication errors also have been reported in prescribing *Celebrex*, a nonsteroidal anti-inflammatory drug for arthritis; *Cerebyx*, an anticonvulsant; and *Celexa*, an antidepressant. It's not hard to see how these names can be confused. In one case, a physician wrote a prescription for *Celexa 200 mg*. But because the antidepressant drug is available in only 20 and 40 milligram doses, the doctor was called and he corrected his prescription to the intended *Celebrex 200 mg*.

In another instance, a pharmacist picked the wrong computer code when he was filling a prescription for a patient who was leaving the hospital. The prescription was for *trovafloxacin 200 mg*, an antibiotic used to treat serious bacterial infections, but the code for *troglitazone 200 mg* came up. Troglitazone is a diabetes drug that has since been withdrawn from the market. The patient found the mistake several days later, when told by a friend that troglitazone is not meant to treat an infection, which is what she had.

The *Pittsburgh Post-Gazette* reported the story of a sixty-seven-year-old woman who was hospitalized for two days after falling in her Pittsburgh apartment.[2] She lived alone and after she fell, she crawled across her apartment to her bedroom, where she went to sleep. Her daughter called her the next morning and came over to drive her mother to the hospital. Her doctor determined that the woman's fall was likely the result of an incorrectly filled prescription he had given her a few days earlier. Instead of receiving a drug for a urinary tract infection, the pharmacy mistakenly dispensed an antidepressant with a similar-sounding name. She already had a separate prescription for 25 mg of the antidepressant, and with the error, she was taking 325 mg of the medication. It's no wonder that she was falling down. We just hope she was sitting down when she received her hospital bill for $4,627.08—which raises the question of who should pay the bill.

Different drugs can also have similar packaging, which can lead to mistakes when they are dispensed. The U.S. Pharmacopeia noted that pharmacists discovered a problem with the similarity of the packaging of *Detrol 1 mg* and *Detrol 2 mg*, a treatment for overactive bladder. The pills for both strengths of the drug looked the same—white, round, and the same size. Pharmacists said that the packaging labels were hard to read and the print could be rubbed off, making it impossible to know the strength of the pill being dispensed. The manufacturer of the drug changed the packaging so the dosage of the pills is easier to read.

By Their Own Hand

Patients can bear severe consequences when the right drug is dispensed but at the wrong dose. But so, too, do family members who unknowingly give from their own hand medication that is dispensed at the wrong dose, leading to the death of their loved one.

This happened to Claudie, a retired sixty-seven-year-old veteran from Kentucky, and his daughter Sandy. Claudie had been diagnosed with a blood clot in his leg at the VA hospital in Lexington. Sandy recalls how her dad was prescribed heparin, which is used to prevent harmful blood clots from forming in the blood vessels. For more than a year, Sandy, the youngest of four children, lovingly and dutifully gave her dad two injections every day, one at 7:30 in the morning and another at 7:30 at night. She says, "We had to rearrange our whole life. I have two children, work forty hours a week, and was going to school."

On a visit to the hospital for a checkup, Claudie was given a prescription for a refill of the heparin. When Claudie and Sandy picked up the prescription at the pharmacy, they noticed that instead of getting small vials labeled 10,000 units, this time they got a larger bottle labeled 1,000 units. Sandy called the hospital after hours to find out if she was supposed to give her dad the same amount of the medication from the larger bottle that she had been giving him from the smaller vials, but couldn't reach anyone. Soon after, when the home health nurse came to the house,

Claudie showed her the medication. She didn't say anything, so he assumed it was okay to take it as he had been all along.

About two months later, Sandy's sister, who had been with Claudie one evening, said that he was having trouble breathing, couldn't get up, and was seeing things that "weren't there." Sandy called the VA right away and was told to bring Claudie in. They drove an hour and a half to the hospital. By the time they arrived, he could hardly breathe and was put on a ventilator. Claudie died three days later from a pulmonary embolism—a blood clot in the lung. The cause of death was the error made when the pharmacy refilled the prescription for heparin at only one-tenth of the dosage he needed to prevent blood clots from forming.

Deadly errors are made in local pharmacies, too. A five-year-old boy's mother knows this firsthand. She went to a pharmacy in Virginia to pick up a prescription for imipramine for her son who had a bed-wetting problem. A pharmacy technician reportedly filled the prescription at five times the intended dose. After the prescription was filled, it was to be checked by the licensed pharmacist on duty. But when the boy's mother came in to pick up the prescription, a clerk removed it from where it was stored, and gave it to her without informing the pharmacist. When the mother returned home, she gave her son two teaspoons of the medication, and the next morning she found him dead. The pharmacy's system of safety checks failed to work as intended to prevent mistakes such as this one.

This tragedy illustrates that unlike other medical mistakes, medication errors can affect family members in profound ways. Both Sandy and the mother of the five-year-old Virginia boy unknowingly gave the wrong medication to their loved ones from their own hand. As Sandy says, "I was feeling so much guilt."

How common are mistakes made at local drug stores? About 2 percent to 3 percent of prescriptions filled have mistakes, based on studies of prescriptions that have been filled but not yet picked up by customers; others say the figure may be as high as 5 percent.

Fortunately the consequences are not always deadly. But the harm is untold. With almost 3 billion prescriptions filled in retail pharmacies each year, and using the 3 percent error rate, this is equivalent to *90 million medication mistakes every year!* In Massachusetts alone, about 2.4 million prescriptions are filled improperly each year, according to a separate study, and almost 90 percent of these mistakes occurred when the customers were given the wrong drug, or the right drug but at the wrong strength.[3]

Sometimes pharmacies dispense the completely wrong drug, which is what happened to a forty-year-old woman with HIV, whose experience was described in an article in the *Journal of the American Medical Association.*[4] She phoned her clinic to request that refills of two prescription drugs be called into a large chain pharmacy. When she picked up the medications, she realized that they were the wrong medications. Instead of getting the antiretroviral medication she needed to treat her HIV infection, she received a tranquilizer and an ulcer medication. She called her doctor immediately to have the mistake corrected. It turns out that when the clinic called the pharmacy, an inexperienced pharmacy technician apparently transcribed the order incorrectly. In response to this mistake, the clinic staff member who calls in a prescription now asks the pharmacist or technician to repeat the name of the drug, the dose, and the mode of administration. This "readout" policy is used by the airline industry to ensure accurate communication. Even better, a year later, the woman noted that every prescription she gets is printed by a computer—none is handwritten. The clinic is still working to set up a system that will electronically transmit prescriptions directly to the pharmacy, which will avoid human error in the transcribing of a refill request, as happened in her case.

Right Drug, Wrong Patient

Once prescription drugs are prescribed and filled, the next challenge is to ensure they are given to the right patient. For a man from suburban New York, they weren't. Tony describes how his dad received the wrong medication while hospitalized after a car accident. "When he was in the hospital, Dad had a nurse who was very funny, he just lit up the room when he came in, and Dad really liked him." The patient sharing the hospital room was diabetic, and one day the nurse gave Tony's dad the medicine meant for his roommate in the other bed. "Dad became unresponsive and went into a coma," Tony says of his father, a former professional boxer and county highway department worker. Shortly afterward, the hospital called the family into the office and said that the nurse had given the wrong medication.

"Dad came out of the coma, but he was a different person," Tony recalls. "That was the beginning of the end. He was never the same. His memory was shot. He used to take his own medicine, but after that, Mom or I had to give it to him four times a day because he could no longer do it himself." When asked what his dad's reaction was when he heard about the mistake, Tony says, "My dad was so easygoing, and he liked the guy [the nurse]. Dad just shrugged his shoulders and said, 'I guess he made a mistake.'" The hospital suggested that the family call an attorney, but they didn't. The family knew the mistake was not intentional, the hospital didn't try to hide it, and the hospital staff apologized. Tony ends the story by saying, "Dad was later diagnosed with Alzheimer's and he lived for four more years. He died in June 2002."

"How Do I Take This Stuff?"

Patients and family members, too, can make mistakes when taking or administering drugs. Many mistakes are made at home because patients are not properly instructed in how to use the medications prescribed.

A man with asthma was prescribed medication that was to be used with an inhaler, which would help him breathe during an asthma attack. The medication wasn't working—not because he wasn't responding to the medication, but because he had not been taught how to use it correctly. The man described how his doctor had demonstrated the use of the inhaler by just holding it in the air and releasing several puffs. So the patient did the same. Thinking it would work better in a confined space, he went out to his car, released two puffs of the medication, and breathed it in.[5] The use of any type of medicine delivery system that's new to a patient should be *clearly demonstrated or explained* by the prescribing clinician. Imagine if this man had experienced a life-threatening asthma attack. The inhaler would have been of no use because he had been *instructed incorrectly* on how to use it.

In another instance of poor physician instruction, a daughter called the doctor's office to say that her mother's constipation was not being relieved. She asked whether her mother could take a different medicine because her mom didn't like the "bitter-tasting, bullet-shaped stuff in the hard-to-open foil." The nurse patiently explained how the suppositories should be used.[6] Fortunately, the incorrect use of this medication caused no harm to the woman.

The Cost of Medication Mistakes

A study published in the *Journal of the American Medical Association* found that almost 2 percent of all patients admitted to two teaching hospitals experienced a medication mistake.[7] Patients who were affected by the errors remained in the hospital an average of four days longer, at a cost of $4,700 per patient. Nationally, this means that an extra $2 billion is spent each year because of medication errors made in hospitals. These estimates do not include the financial costs borne by patients after they go home.

Nor do they account for the human costs that medication mistakes can impose on patients and their families. Prescription drugs are powerful chemical entities and, as you have seen, can be so easily misused. For as much good as they can do, they can do so much harm when used improperly and without care. Patti, whom you met earlier, watched her mother die from an overdose of morphine in the hospital. She describes the impact this error had on her. "After my mother died, I was going to school, which was located right near the hospital. I drove to school every day for nine months and saw that hospital every time. I would spend the second half hour of the trip crying in the car and trying to compose myself before going to class. My hope is gone, my faith is gone, and my trust is gone."

■ ■ ■

As the story of the nine-month-old in the beginning of this chapter shows, even infants are not immune from errors. Because their small bodies are less able to handle medication errors, they can suffer more serious consequences. Critically ill infants in neonatal intensive care units are especially at risk, compared with more healthy neonates and older children. A study published in the *Journal of the American Medical Association* reported the number of medication errors among 10,000 medication orders filled for children in two large hospitals.[8] Of these orders, 616 mistakes occurred, which is about 6 percent of the medication orders. Twenty-six of these mistakes harmed a child in some fashion. If any more good reason is needed to prevent medication mistakes, think of the children.

part three

The Silent White Line

8 | A Culture of Coverup

We know from the writings of ancient Greek physicians who practiced medicine more than two thousand years ago that some errors occurred because physicians lacked the knowledge and technical skills to render the proper care to their patients. These same reasons remain the cause of some of the errors made in medicine today.

Meanwhile, another recognizable characteristic of the profession has been carried down through the generations. The prevailing ethic noted in the ancient texts was not to disclose errors to the patient. According to Dr. Steven Miles, "In the dozens of accounts of errors in the ancient Greek texts, none advocates or illustrates telling the patient or a relative about the error."[1] And so it remains today.

The patients and families whom you have met have all experienced this handed-down tradition of nondisclosure—a tradition that by now has worn thin and must be discarded. It manifests itself in the wall of silence that these people came up against at different points along their journey in the health system: when trying to find information to help them choose a good doctor, when trying to understand what went wrong when a medical mistake occurred, and when seeking accountability in the aftermath of a mistake.

From Behind the Wall of Silence

The culture of coverup in the medical profession has deep roots and extends beyond the borders of nations. In England in July 2000, an inquiry was conducted to investigate excessive mortality rates among children under one year of age who had heart operations at the Bristol Royal Infirmary, a teaching hospital associated with Bristol University's Medical School. During the inquiry, reference was made to the "club culture" that prevailed in which a physician's progress up the hierarchy depended not on performance but on whether there was a "fit" within the club. Those who challenged the status quo and questioned whether the clinical outcomes for patients were as good as they should be were viewed as disloyal. Rather than embrace a critical assessment of performance and patient care, the club exacted a high price for this disloyalty— ostracism from the club. This club culture was the mortar in the wall of silence that, in this case, led to surgeries being performed whose resulting mortality rates were double that of mortality rates of other facilities—in sum, unnecessary deaths of children and devastated parents.

The wall of silence in medicine is little different from the "blue line" in police departments that encourages members of the "tribe" to close ranks to protect their own. Many doctors are willing participants and do not report colleagues whose practice of medicine is substandard and a danger to the health of patients.

Donna found this to be true when caring for her mother, Madeline, whose failed hip surgery was ignored by her orthopedic surgeon. Donna recalls the surgeon who came to repair the damage as saying he wouldn't report the poor care provided by his colleague because he didn't want to go against his peers.

Similarly, Justin's mom, Carey, remembers a physician who was willing to come forward as an expert witness in the case of her son, who died after a life-threatening condition was misdiagnosed. The expert witness backed out when he found out that the doctor who missed the diagnosis had been one of his students.

Meanwhile, conscientious physicians tell stories, privately, of their peers who are providing poor care to patients or practicing unethically; if these physicians speak up, they are accused of being arrogant and threatened with retribution. If they try to bring quality concerns up the line, they are accused of not being a team player. Their jobs could be at risk.

Here's what one health care provider wrote to us: "I have crossed that line, the white wall of silence, that puts me in the unenviable position of being subject to scrutiny and dismissal at any time. Addressing the issues openly as I have makes people nervous, and they worry that I may be a liability, a person who is not a 'team player' or, in other words, one who is not willing to cover up for the company team at any cost."

One Boston physician conducted a study at the hospital where he works that documented the number of patients who suffered cardiac arrests as a result of suboptimal responses by physicians to clinical signs and symptoms. He says, "My junior colleagues and I wrote up the findings and submitted a paper to the *New England Journal of Medicine* for their review, sending it also along to the chair of medicine in my department. I was driving home that day and was paged. I recognized the number as his. When I called him back, he told me he was furious, and that I couldn't submit the paper with the findings describing the problems at our hospital. He also said I had to do the study all over again, which I did over the next couple of years. I got the same findings. He could say little more. I submitted the paper to the *Journal of the American Medical Association,* and they published it, along with an editorial congratulating us for having the courage to be forthright. I can't prove it, but I suspect my appointment to full professor was delayed for several years as a result of this paper."

As a profession, medicine has relied on peer review to ensure the quality of care its members provide. Peer review is a self-regulating function in which physicians evaluate their colleagues and hold them accountable, a distinguishing feature of the profession.

But when the conscientious physicians are silenced, peer review breaks down and patients bear the brunt of the poor quality care that is tolerated, as in the following case.

A physician in New York had his license revoked permanently on several charges of gross negligence. Prior to that, his former physician colleagues, who spoke to a *New York Times* reporter on the condition of anonymity, said that the physician's problems were quite well known at the hospital where they all practiced. The physicians even discouraged doctors in training from working with him, but they apparently didn't discourage unsuspecting patients from being treated by him.

Kept in the Dark

When deciding which doctor to entrust one's life to, doing your homework can really pay off—but not always. Judy, a woman from California, had done her homework to learn more about doctors who could perform a face lift and liposuction. As reported on *Nightline*, she contacted the Medical Board of California to check her doctor's background. The board-certified plastic surgeon she had selected had a clear record. But during the ten-hour procedure, her blood was so diluted with liposuction fluid that a coroner ruled she had bled to death. The doctor and the anesthesiologist both lost their licenses after the medical board concluded they had been negligent.

It was too late for Judy, though. She didn't know that the doctor she'd chosen had at least three previous malpractice lawsuits filed against him in another state. Nor did she know that there is a national data bank that contains this information about doctors' backgrounds and malpractice history. This information is off-limits to the public because the medical profession lobbied to keep the information secret from the public view. Her husband told *Nightline* that if he and his wife had had access to that information, he believed that his wife would be alive today.

THE NATIONAL PRACTITIONER DATA BANK

In the 1980s, pressure was building to give the public more protection against incompetent doctors. Then-Representative Ron Wyden of Oregon, a sponsor of the proposed legislation, noted the following in an Op-Ed piece in the *Washington Post* in 1986. "The House Energy and Commerce Health and Environment Subcommittee heard testimony indicating that three to five percent of the doctors in this country account for most of the malpractice. The need for legislation is clear. There is no effective national system for keeping tabs on doctors who are truly incompetent. Physicians have told the health subcommittee on which I sit that they are now afraid to speak out when a colleague malpractices. Hospitals can't take actions against physicians they know are incompetent because they fear the legal consequences. The result: the incompetent doctor continues to practice, inflicting poor care and soaring costs on the unsuspecting."

In 1986, Congress established the National Practitioner Data Bank as a central clearinghouse for information about doctors and other health professionals. It is the country's only national source of information on adverse actions taken against physicians, dentists, and other health professionals, and it was not accessible to Judy and her husband and remains inaccessible today.

The data bank does not contain information on medical mistakes but does include information on whether health professionals have been named in a medical malpractice settlement. It also has records of disciplinary actions taken by state licensing boards, including revocation or suspension of a medical license and probationary status of a license. Disciplinary actions taken by a hospital, such as the revocation of a health professional's hospital privileges, are noted as well.

The data bank has reports on approximately 193,000 health professionals, and almost 133,000 of them are physicians. Most have just one report, and it is usually a report on a malpractice claim that was paid. The information in the data bank is not perfect and may contain duplicate reports on a single disciplinary action. Those who have been reported to the data bank can dispute the accuracy of the information in it, although inaccurate information is not always corrected. Just as Americans want to ensure that their credit report contains accurate information, doctors and other health care professionals want reports about them in the data bank to be accurate—not an impossible task.

Early versions of the legislation allowed the public to have access to the information, but lobbying by the American Medical Association led Congress to *drop the provision granting public access.* Opponents of public access say that malpractice information can be misunderstood by the public, who will assume that because a doctor has malpractice settlements, he or she is a bad doctor. In fairness to good doctors, a malpractice settlement does not necessarily mean that a doctor is incompetent or negligent. It may simply mean that the insurance company chose to settle a nuisance complaint rather than bear the cost of prolonged legal proceedings. Nonetheless, people who have witnessed medical mistakes firsthand want this information easily available to help them make an informed decision when selecting a doctor. By keeping this information secret, patients and families have to do their homework without the textbook that would help them do it best.

Tony, whose Dad was given the wrong medication and went into a coma, was witness to yet another medical mistake. He wishes he could have had access to information in the national data bank because it would have helped him and his family make a better decision when selecting a doctor for his mother. Tony's mother, Eleanor, went into the hospital to have her gall bladder removed. The doctor punctured her bile duct, and bile leaked out of the duct and into her body cavity. Tony recalls, "We finally found a doctor who repairs bile ducts. He just shook his head and said a lot of doctors are not familiar with the use of a laser and they do damage to the bile duct. He basically made a new bile duct and Mom needs to be monitored twice a year.

"I wrote a letter to the original doctor telling him what happened, and he never answered. He probably just threw it in the garbage. Then I found out you can go to the county courthouse to look up a doctor's name and see if there are any malpractice judgments. I went with someone who helped me, and we found that Mom's first doctor had been through three malpractice settlements. As we were going through the records and reading what had happened to other patients, my friend said, 'What a butcher!' Mom didn't want to sue since she came from the old school, grew up in Brooklyn, and just wanted to get better."

NOT LIVING UP TO THE LAW

Hospitals are required by law to check with the data bank when doctors apply for privileges to take care of patients at a hospital. They also are required to check every two years with the data bank as part of ongoing review of the physicians who have privileges. In 1999, more than 3.5 million information requests were made to the data bank, more than four times the number in 1991.

The data bank is an effective information tool only if hospitals and other health care organizations actually report adverse actions involving a health care professional. Federal law requires this information to be reported. But hospitals are not complying. Since the data bank was established, more than 60 percent of hospitals have never reported any adverse action. It was expected that hospitals would report more than 1,000 disciplinary actions every month, yet fewer than 1,000 are reported in a year.

Managed care organizations aren't much better. From September 1, 1990, to September 30, 1999, they reported only 715 adverse events to the data bank. Eighty-four percent of them have never reported any adverse action. The investigative arm of the federal Department of Health and Human Services, the Office of the Inspector General, notes that, "With close to 100 million individuals enrolled in these organizations and hundreds of thousands of physicians and dentists associated with them, fewer than 1,000 adverse action reports over nearly a decade serves for all practical purposes as 'nonreporting.'" What's the reason? The Inspector General's office says that many managed care plans give modest attention to oversight. They rely on the hospitals and medical groups they contract with to do the reporting and state licensure boards to monitor the quality of care provided by health professionals. But medical groups are saddled with the same problem as hospitals—they don't want to expose their poor-performing colleagues.

INSIDER INFORMATION

Doctors and nurses know colleagues whom they wouldn't want caring for them or their spouses or their friends. Nurses know which doctors are competent and communicate well with patients. Pharmacists know which doctors write legibly and prescribe correctly. Doctors know the reputations of their colleagues and see firsthand the care they provide when they cover for them on weekends. Both doctors and nurses know which hospitals—and which units—are well staffed by good nurses.

When doctors or nurses have a family member or friend who needs medical care, they call their fellow health care professionals to find out which doctors are good and which to avoid. This grapevine is an effective and efficient way of obtaining accurate information about the skill and competence of a physician and which hospitals are well staffed enough to perform certain procedures.

But most Americans are not privy to this insider information and have only inadequate information to make critical decisions about choosing a doctor. Here is what one nurse wrote to her colleagues in a nursing journal: "Think about it; your neighbor needs coronary bypass surgery and plans to have it at nearby Hospital A.

You know that this hospital performs less than five of these procedures per week and is fraught with internal political struggles. The surgeon is known to be a poor communicator. The hospital has trouble attracting the best nurses, and relies heavily on agency staff. What do you do? Keep quiet, let the neighbor have the surgery, even though the teaching hospital twenty miles away has a far better reputation across the board? Hopefully not. You will probably gently, and perhaps then not so delicately, urge your friend to at least get a second opinion. If nurses can do this level of quality assurance for their loved ones, shouldn't we at the very least be trying to do this for our communities?"[2]

Coverup at the Bedside

The culture of coverup also manifests itself at the bedside when mistakes occur. Ockie's daughter, Rebecca, recalls, "While my dad was in the hospital, we requested a family meeting with the doctors—they didn't offer it. We wanted to understand what happened to our father. The risk manager was there, the head of nursing, the anesthesiologist, and others. Prior to the meeting, we were told point-blank that we should not waste the physicians' time in the meeting asking about the [nasogastric tube] incident, which eventually led to our father's death. At the time we were very vulnerable and emotional. It was in the back of our minds that if we made them angry, it could jeopardize the care our dad would get. We are a very vocal family, but they put you in such a position that you can't question. They intimidated us. It's as if we, the family, did something wrong."

Pursuing Justice Without Success

Patients and their families also encounter the wall of silence when they seek to hold someone justly accountable for the all the immeasurable harm they bear. With her daughter's help, Madeline did all the right things an educated consumer should do to raise her concern about the poor care she received when she broke her hip. She wrote to the hospital expressing her dissatisfaction. The hospital wrote back saying "there were no deficiencies in care. Unfortunately, sometimes complications can occur post-surgery which are not related to any deficiencies in care."

Madeline then wrote to the Joint Commission on Accreditation of Healthcare Organizations and it responded saying that they give "serious consideration to all issues that may reflect noncompliance with Joint Commission standards and we appreciate your providing us this information. We have updated our database for this organization (the hospital where the first surgery took place) to reflect your concerns. We will monitor the organization for patterns of care over time in the area of your concern."

Still not satisfied, she wrote to her state's medical board, which investigates complaints about physicians whose actions may cause harm to the public. The case was presented to the board for its review. The board found insufficient evidence "to support the prosecution of the allegation that a violation had occurred."

The result is that no one was held accountable for the poor care Madeline received. No one knows—or cares to find out—whether her experience was a one-time aberration for the doctor who did not recognize that the first surgery failed, and thus caused her excruciating pain, or whether a pattern of complications exists in his care of patients. No corrective steps were taken to prevent other older patients from suffering similar consequences of negligence. Future patients who come to see him—even if they do their homework and contact the state medical board—will never know that at least one complaint was filed with the state medical board because medical boards keep this information confidential. No one will know that Madeline probably would have died from the negligence of a licensed physician were it not for the actions of her dedicated daughter.

State Medical Boards: Your Tax Dollars at Work?

A framed medical license, which is granted by the state in which a doctor practices, hangs on the wall of many physicians' offices. This document seemingly provides some tangible reassurance to patients that they are placing their health and their lives in the hands of a skilled and competent professional. Most Americans assume that because a doctor is licensed, some entity is watching to ensure he or she provides high-quality care.

Physicians have to renew their license to practice every several years. But to do so, they only have to fill out a form, pay a fee, and document that they have met continuing medical education requirements. These continuing education requirements can be fulfilled by attending a conference, listening to a presentation, or reading medical literature. To maintain a medical license, doctors' knowledge is not re-examined, and their competence and skills are not reassessed.

Most physicians now, though, are board-certified in a specialty, which means they have been tested for their knowledge in caring for patients with conditions related to their specialty. Doctors can be board-certified in specialties such as internal medicine, obstetrics and gynecology, and pediatrics. Board certification is different from a medical license. A medical license is granted by the state in which the physician practices medicine, while board certification is granted by a specialty board composed of physicians. Periodic recertification demonstrates that a physician has maintained continued qualifications to practice in a certain specialty.

While states do not test physicians as part of license renewal, states are responsible for protecting the public's health and safety by setting standards for the practice of medicine, enforcing those standards, and ensuring that doctors who are licensed are practicing medicine accordingly. In many states, medical-licensing board members are appointed by the governor, often with the blessing of the state medical societies who, with little hesitation, wield their clout during election campaigns.

State medical boards discipline physicians for a host of reasons, including fraudulently billing for services never performed, having sex with a patient, performing unnecessary surgery, prescribing narcotics for their own use, and performing surgery on the wrong part of a patient's body. A review of state medical board disciplinary actions reveals that medical boards are much more likely to discipline a physician for abuse of drugs or alcohol than for care that doesn't meet a quality standard the public would expect.

But state medical boards discipline doctors only if they are informed about substandard practices. Boards are rarely proactive and only if the media has uncovered an egregious case of misconduct by a physician. If a physician is dismissed from a hospital because of practices that endanger patients, the hospital may not necessarily notify the state medical board. To avoid a confrontation with a doctor, and even a lawsuit, the hospital may just let the doctor quietly resign. The same doctor can go to work at another hospital, with no record that he or she potentially or actually endangered a patient, and the state medical board can't take any disciplinary action if it is not reported. The lesson here is that the state medical license hanging on the wall in the doctor's office may not always be a "Good Housekeeping Seal of Approval."

Meanwhile, many members of the public are eager to—and do—contact the medical board in their state to report concerns about a physician's incompetent or negligent care. Yet these complaints virtually always end up nowhere. Every person you met in Chapter 2 who has sought redress from a state medical board, along with others with whom we have spoken, gave the same response when asked about the impact of their efforts: "Just useless." Diana, who suffered egregiously for many years from poor care and provided documentation of negligence to her state's medical board, reflects on her experience this way, "The medical boards are useless—useless to the public; they are quite 'useful' to the doctors who hide behind their findings. It's like having the fox patrolling the henhouse."

FOXES PATROLLING THE HENHOUSE

It is very hard for the lay person to understand how medical boards allow some physicians to continue to practice medicine. A doctor in Virginia was found guilty in federal court of unlawful sexual conduct with a patient and was sentenced to a month in jail. According to state records, it took two years for the medical board to notify the physician that his license to practice would be placed on probation and that he must complete fifty hours of continuing medical education and undergo a psychiatric evaluation. Even though his license was restricted, he was still authorized to see patients, with the provision that a chaperon be present for all physical exams of women and of children under the age of eighteen. The medical board wrote to the physician a year later stating that he complied with all the terms set out by the board, that his license to practice medicine was no longer restricted, and that he no longer needed a chaperon when conducting physical exams.

It is hard to imagine any husband who would want his wife to be treated by a doctor convicted of sexual misconduct or any father who would want his daughter to be examined by someone with such a record. But how would they know? The answer is they won't. Local newspapers often report on food establishments that receive citations from the local health department for unsanitary practices or serving spoiled food. But there is no comparable reporting to inform the public when doctors are allowed to continue to treat patients after being convicted of such a crime.

As one observer who has watched his state medical board very closely said, "They give licenses to convicted criminals." He cites the records of the medical board meetings in his state in which the board granted a license to a physician who had been convicted of fraud and lost his medical license in New York, a state whose medical board is more stringent than boards in other states.

How can these actions be explained when they are so contrary to a layperson's sense of justice and common sense? At best, there is a chasm between state medical boards' views and the beliefs of concerned citizens when it comes to determining whether a person's character is deserving of a license to practice medicine.

The wife of a seventy-seven-year-old retired Sears store manager, who came within inches of death because of substandard care, said, "I think there are separate laws for these people. It's not that we are anti-doctor. Both my husband and I have brothers in the medical profession."

We know a retired pilot who served in World War II who has been unsuccessful in obtaining any redress after bringing complaints to a state medical board after having a personal experience with medical error. He reflects on the difference between aviation and health care this way: "When a plane crashes, it isn't the local pilots' union that comes to investigate the cause of the crash. They aren't judged by the old boys' club. It's the National Transportation Safety Board and the Federal Aviation Administration who conduct the investigation."

MONEY MAKES A BLIND EYE

After a physician is disciplined, too often it is business as usual. An investigation by the *New York Times* of the records of doctors who were disciplined by New York's Office of Professional Medical Conduct revealed disturbing findings.[3] The disciplinary records were matched with hospital admitting records. More than 75 percent of doctors who were disciplined for negligence over a period of eight years went back to work practicing medicine right after they were sanctioned by the state. Hospitals seemed especially eager to hire doctors with a record of negligent care if they admitted a large volume of patients and generated revenue for the hospital.

Some hospitals hide behind a state's licensing practices to protect themselves. If the state does not revoke the license of a physician, they assume that the doctor must still be fit to care for patients. Other hospitals are proactive and don't wait until a physician's license is revoked to deny him or her access to patients. Can

any hospital that hires doctors who perform egregious acts of negligence have the interests of its patients as its top priority?

One of the most startling cases of failed oversight is that of an
obstetrician who practiced at a hospital in New York City. After
successfully delivering a baby girl by cesarean section, he carved
his initials in the mother's abdomen using a surgical scalpel. The
nurses watched in horror as he did it. According to state health
department records, the doctor surrendered his medical license,
but it took five months for him to do so. The state health department reportedly fined the hospital $14,000 for failing to ade-
quately monitor the physician when earlier complaints were made
against him by hospital staff. The patient filed a lawsuit against the
physician and reportedly received a $1.75 million settlement.

The revelations in New York came at a time when the state
health commissioner, Dr. Antonia C. Novello, was publicizing the
hospitals and doctors who provide incompetent care. Quoted in
the *New York Times*, Novello said she intends to keep such doctors
unemployed, stating, "When you break the trust of public good, I
don't think you should be able to practice."[4]

What the Public Can Do

The public is becoming more sophisticated about gathering information to make informed decisions about many aspects of their
lives. Thanks to the Internet, many Americans are more knowledgeable than ever about investing in stocks and mutual funds.
While the downturn in the stock market has caused people to lose
money, no one is suggesting that financial information be made
unavailable to the public. On the contrary, in the wake of the
Enron and WorldCom scandals, Congress is requiring companies
to make more information available to the public, not less.

Meanwhile, millions of Americans use the Internet to obtain
information about their health; if they have an illness they scour
the Internet to learn about treatment options. But when it comes

to one of the most important decisions Americans make—the selection of a physician to care for them—the medical profession keeps this information out of the hands of the people who need it most.

"TRUST BUT VERIFY"

What is the public to do when many hospitals and other health facilities haven't taken the necessary steps to ensure that poorly performing professionals are prevented from treating patients? The system says, "Trust us." But that doesn't work anymore. The system is losing the public's trust, and it has to work fast to regain it.

You'll remember Daniel, the former White House official whose medically induced disability brought an end to a brilliant career. His advice to people who are anticipating using the health care system is, "Trust but verify," referring to Ronald Reagan's advice about dealing with the Russians.

SEEK OUT STATE WEB SITES

While it is unlikely that the federal government will give the public access to the National Practitioner Data Bank in the foreseeable future, state governments are slowly beginning to meet the public's demand for information about doctors. Many states now have Web sites that give profiles of physicians licensed to practice there.

Massachusetts has mounted one of the more comprehensive initiatives to help its residents make informed decisions about the doctors they select—with the leadership and active involvement of the Massachusetts Medical Society, the publisher of the *New England Journal of Medicine*. The state Board of Registration in Medicine compiles profiles of each physician licensed in the state that include information on the educational background of the physician, criminal convictions, actions by hospitals to restrict privileges, and disciplinary actions taken by Massachusetts and other state medical boards such as license suspension, revocation, or reinstatement. Malpractice information is available, too, along with information on whether a certain number of malpractice settlements is typical for a physician in a particular specialty such as obstetrics, which is more susceptible to malpractice claims than other specialties. This information is available on the Internet (www.massmedboard.org) and through a toll-free telephone number.

The Massachusetts Web site is popular, and since it was set up in 1996, it has had more than 7 million visitors. Press releases summarizing disciplinary actions taken against named doctors are issued monthly by the board and posted on the Web site. Here are some examples of the disciplinary actions taken: a physician's license was suspended for allegedly attacking a friend with a baseball bat, causing him serious bodily harm; a physician's license was suspended when he was convicted in a court of indecent assault and battery of patients; a physician's license was revoked after he was found guilty in a court of first-degree murder; a physician was placed on probation because he had been disciplined by another state medical board after being arrested for allegedly using illegal drugs; a physician resigned when the Board investigated his failure to notify it that he had been disciplined in at least four other states. He had licenses to practice in three additional states.

The California medical board also issues press releases (see www.medbd.ca.gov) when disciplinary actions are taken against physicians. One such example: a physician who was ordered to surrender his medical license for gross negligence. He allowed medical assistants to perform tests without physician supervision, and he interpreted tests when he was not competent to do so. Another physician was required to surrender his license when he reportedly put illegal drugs into drinks he prepared for female patients without their knowledge or consent and had inappropriate sexual contact with patients.

High-profile cases of egregious conduct by some physicians in New York state, along with strong advocacy by consumer groups, prompted the state to make information on doctors licensed to practice in New York accessible to the public. In February 2002, the state launched a Web site—www.nydoctorprofile.com—that provides information on physicians including professional and community activities, criminal records, actions taken by other states' medical boards, malpractice judgments, hospital practice restrictions, and education and training background. This Web site links to the state's Office of Professional Medical Conduct Web site, which reports disciplinary actions taken against a physician (www.health.state.ny.us/nysdoh/opmc/main.htm). The disciplinary actions can be searched by the name of the physician. Anyone can register to receive an e-mail message when new reports of disciplinary actions are posted.

Virginia's Web site with physician profiles (www.vahealth-providers.com) has information about the education, location of practice, and disciplinary history of 31,000 doctors licensed to practice in that state. The Web site was launched in July 2001, three years after the state legislature passed a law requiring public disclosure of this information. Unlike the physician profiles on the Massachusetts Web site, which do not include specific details of disciplinary actions (they must be requested in writing), Virginia's Web site includes images of the actual correspondence between the medical board and the physician regarding disciplinary actions. This information helps the reader know exactly why a physician was disciplined.

TELLING THE PUBLIC THE TRUTH

The progress these and other states have made in disclosing valuable information to the public is laudable and indicates that, at least in some states, the voices of consumers are being heard. Yet states need to make greater strides if they want to provide the public with the information they need to make informed decisions. There are some pretty big gaps in the information that states are providing. Some have no detailed physician profiles on the Internet—the easiest and most accessible way to report this information to the public. On many of the Web sites, information about disciplinary actions taken by the boards is hard to find. A loophole is that physician profiles are mostly self-reported, and the states say they don't have the money to verify them for accuracy, so the information may not be complete or accurate. Many states' physician profiles don't contain information on disciplinary actions and other adverse actions taken by other states' medical boards, yet many physicians have had a license to practice in several states. A physician in Virginia didn't tell the state medical board that he had been sanctioned by as many as six other states. It isn't practical for consumers to search the Web sites of every state medical board—assuming this information is even accessible online.

The Federation of State Medical Boards, which is the association of individual state medical boards, has taken a step in the right direction. Its Web site (www.docinfo.org) gives the public access to background and disciplinary information about physicians in all fifty states. Yet it doesn't have information about medical malpractice settlements or actions by hospitals to restrict a physician's privileges—both of which are recorded in the National Practitioner Data Bank.

■ ■ ■

Having a national data bank be accessible to the public is the only way patients and families will have the tools to make informed decisions. Even the Federation of State Medical Boards realizes this when it says on its Web site, "This information is essential to your safety and well-being and will help you make better and more informed decisions about your physicians."

But Congress so far has failed to act and give the public access to the already existing National Practitioner Data Bank. It's just a matter of time, however, before medical special interest groups lose the fight to keep this information secret. The Internet age is making access to information a way of life. And now, access to information about doctors is no longer just an issue about the doctors. It's about the safety of patients and families who want to know—and have a right to know—the track record of the people in whom they place their trust. The longer valuable information is kept secret, the more the public will think there is something to hide.

Contrary to what the naysayers would have legislators believe, the sky hasn't fallen with the release of information about disciplinary actions and malpractice judgments. The naysayers underestimate the public's ability to use information in a responsible way. Even if the public knows the information exists—and most do not—individuals are likely to use it as just one source, combined with other information, to make more informed decisions about their health care.

In a 1948 speech to the New York State Publishers Association, Arthur Hays Sulzberger, the publisher of the *New York Times* from 1935 to 1963, said, "Obviously a man's judgment cannot be better than the information on which he has based it. Give him the truth and he may still go wrong when he has the chance to be right, but give him no news or present him only with distorted and incomplete data...and you destroy his whole reasoning process, and make him something less of a man."

9 | Don't Ask, Don't Tell

"I'm turning fifty next month and my wife is urging me to have a colonoscopy. I've been asking around about who to go to. My friends have given me a couple of names of doctors, but where can I find out how many of these things they've done and which doctors have patients that end up with more complications? And how do you know whether it's just normal complications or really the guy just doesn't do it very well?"

"My doctor says I need to have a procedure done soon, maybe next month. Am I at more or less risk of having something go wrong if I have it done in the hospital across town where I have to spend the night, or should I have it done at an outpatient surgical facility not too far from my house—where I can get in and out quickly?"

"My daughter needs to be hospitalized. Do children suffer from medical mistakes more or less than adults?"

The answer to all these excellent questions is, "No one knows." The wall of silence manifests itself yet again and denies the American public access to basic and vital information when they are putting their life in someone's hands.

No one knows which hospitals or surgical centers might be especially fertile breeding grounds for medical errors and which do an exemplary job keeping errors to a minimum. We don't know how often the wrong limbs are amputated or procedures are performed on the wrong patient—even though these are easily identifiable and measurable errors. Experts believe that these types of events are rare, but no one knows how rare.

This information isn't available because health care facilities are not required to report such events, they don't want to report it, and fight tooth and nail to keep the wall of silence firmly intact. Nobody asks, and nobody tells. Meanwhile, in our collective infinite wisdom, insurance companies and government programs, including Medicare and Medicaid, continue to pay the bills for care provided as the result of errors, which further lulls hospitals and other health care organizations into complacency.

The IOM committee recommended nationwide mandatory reporting of errors by hospitals to state governments when those errors result in serious injury or death. Not surprisingly, these recommendations have come up against a solid wall of resistance from the hospital industry.

Contagious Complacency

As in many aspects of life, if we don't measure a problem—and don't want to measure it—we aren't serious about fixing it. In other sectors of our economy, when the health of the public is at stake, a different approach is used.

Consider for a moment how other threats to the public's health are handled. When mad cow disease came to be known in England in the 1980s, the importance of a safe food supply and the government's role in ensuring its safety became abundantly clear. Mad cow is an incurable brain disease found in cattle that can be transmitted to humans. About one hundred people, most from Britain, have died apparently from eating meat from infected cattle. The U.S. Department of Agriculture and the meat industry have worked hard to track and prevent any possible outbreaks of mad cow disease on this side of the Atlantic, with the result that American consumers—and cattle—have so far been well protected.

Assume for a minute the hypothetical scenario in which a million people died from contaminated meat in the United States in the last ten years. In response, Congress held hearings, and the President ordered a government-wide task force. At those hearings, members of Congress heard testimony about notable voluntary efforts that a few cattlemen, meatpackers, state and local governments, and grocery stores were taking to ensure that meat was safe to eat. Imagine that food safety and consumer groups urged Congress to establish a national data system to track contaminated meat and find its source, but the meat industry, which was making big campaign contributions to members of Congress, successfully fought those efforts, and no mandatory national tracking system was established. The status quo was maintained, and people continued to die regularly from eating tainted meat.

Imagine that cattlemen and the meat industry reported contaminated meat voluntarily, only when they had the time to or wanted to do so, and kept this information confidential among themselves. They claimed that if they reported incidents of contaminated meat to authorities and the public, people sickened by it would sue them.

Now imagine further that the federal government announced that its major initiative was to fund research to stem the disease, and meanwhile, people were dying every day. In this scenario, grocery stores couldn't identify which meat processing plants were distributing meat that was safe to eat, and they successfully lobbied for immunity from liability if customers sued them. Yet the consumer had no way of knowing which grocery store might be selling contaminated meat.

Medical mistakes and mad cow disease are very different events, but they both can result in human fatalities. Medical mistakes don't spread like disease, and most often they are not discrete, identifiable events that are easy to track or measure. Some errors are obvious—surgery on the wrong person, for example. But when it comes to perforated colons during colonoscopies (a known risk of the procedure), when does a high rate of perforation become error and not just the result of complications? The answer to this question can be subject to legitimate debate among the best doctors, but we don't even know complication rates among different doctors and health care facilities to begin to compare outcomes.

Yet even with these big differences between mad cow disease and medical errors, a commonality exists. Preventing medical errors requires some of the same steps that are taken to tackle any outbreak that threatens our well-being, whether it is tainted meat, the spread of HIV/AIDS, or, more recently, the West Nile virus.

The first step is understanding how prevalent the problem is, identifying and tracking where it is occurring, who is affected, why they were affected, and how. Prevention of future outbreaks requires vigilant monitoring and reporting. If mad cow disease, which can spread so quickly, were detected in the United States, you can be sure the government would take immediate and dramatic steps to eradicate it.

The stakes would be enormous, since an outbreak would threaten the safety of the nation's meat supply, the health of the public, the livelihoods of people working in the industry, and the perception of the United States abroad. The sense of security and trust that Americans have about the safety of the U.S. food supply would be irreparably harmed.

Unlike the approach used to prevent mad cow disease, however, there is no prevailing attitude that medical mistakes, like disease outbreaks, should be as rare as they can possibly be. And while medical mistakes are not contagious, complacent attitudes about them are contagious. This explains why hardly any capacity exists in the public or private sector to track how often errors occur, where and why they occur, and whom they affect.

"The need to systematically build in safety has not achieved a level of urgency in our health care system," says Dennis O'Leary, president of the Joint Commission on Accreditation of Healthcare Organizations. "You need a CEO who says, 'We have a problem here, and I am going to hire some industrial engineers, and we are going to take our system apart and put it back together until it's safe.' " Just as market share and financial performance are top priorities for the boards of trustees of health care organizations, medical mistake tracking needs to be added to their regular agendas.

Mandatory Reporting of Errors

Nor is there any urgency for mandatory reporting of medical mistakes by hospitals and other health care facilities to state governments or other entities that can track the frequency of errors. Is it enough to rely on the voluntary efforts of the dedicated people who are working with urgency to make health care safe in their facilities? No, it isn't. We don't rely on voluntary efforts to stem other causes of large numbers of human fatalities.

Gail Warden, an eminent health care executive and national leader in patient safety, has said, "As soon as we're able to start mandatory reporting of medical mistakes, I think we'll find that medical mistakes get corrected."

Americans have the same opinion. About 70 percent of people surveyed believe that health care organizations should be required to report serious mistakes and to make this information available to the public. Health care executives have a different view. Among those surveyed by the American College of Healthcare Executives, 42 percent of the respondents said they would support a mandatory reporting system for mistakes that result in death or serious injury. Another 42 percent opposed it, and the remaining respondents were undecided. Doctors are the least enthusiastic about reporting errors to state governments. Only 23 percent think it would be very effective.[1]

What is the consequence of medical errors not being reported? The American public will remain in the dark about how many children bleed to death every year after a tonsillectomy or die from medication errors, and how many women mistakenly have double mastectomies because of errors in the handling of biopsy results, to use just a few examples. Without error reporting, we cannot know whether these tragedies, over time, are increasing or decreasing in frequency.

Owning Up to Mistakes

One of the biggest barriers to mandatory reporting of medical mistakes is the difficulty most people have in admitting they have made one. For conscientious people who pride themselves on trying to do everything right—and many doctors and nurses are exceedingly careful in their work, admitting a mistake is one of the hardest things to do. It's even harder to admit a mistake when the environment where they work is one of blame and finger pointing.

A physician was asked about her hospital's new disclosure policy, which now requires doctors to disclose errors to their patients. She says, "Who wants to be the first doctor or nurse to do this? You don't really know until you try it whether the hospital will stand behind you when the mistake was a culmination of errors in the system, or whether there will be repercussions. It's like getting the smallpox vaccine. No one wants to go first. Everyone wants to wait and see how it works on other people."

This perspective is from a physician whose patient was harmed and came close to death because of errors in the system. The physician disclosed the error, explained why it occurred, and rendered an apology. If disclosure is hard for a physician who already practices disclosure, it can be more difficult for others who haven't had the inclination to do so.

Yet, as Elizabeth's mother says, "When things go wrong, this is a test of character. Those who missed the fact that Elizabeth's cancer had come back were the fastest to run." When mistakes occur, it is also a test of character for the health care organization. Does it manage medical mistakes that occur inside its own walls in an ethical manner? Or does it "tuck its tail and figure out how to make itself not responsible," to use the words of Elizabeth's mother.

Drivers who are involved in a motor vehicle accident are required by law to stop and identify themselves and call for assistance if someone is injured. Even if a driver isn't at fault, the law requires him or her to stop. Let's assume it is a rainy, foggy night, and a pedestrian dashes across the road. The driver doesn't see him and hits him. When a driver stops, he or she is admitting that something terrible has happened, whether the driver was at fault or not. The driver might be the subject of an investigation involving the police and insurance companies; he might face a lawsuit and even media attention. Questions might be raised about whether the driver was drinking or taking medication or had an argument with his wife and steamed out of the house. It might be quicker and easier for the driver to keep on going and never stop. But the law requires drivers to respond in an ethical manner.

Physicians are held to a higher standard than people in other professions. Patients who are injured or ill from disease place their lives and their trust in the hands of physicians and expect that, as difficult as it may be, they will be told the truth when a mistake occurs. They expect that medical mistakes will be handled in a moral and ethical manner and they won't be abandoned. When the people whom you met encountered the exact opposite, their anger began to build.

"Never Events"

Currently, only twenty states require health care facilities to report medical mistakes; several others have voluntary reporting. The states' reporting initiatives are well-intended efforts, yet only six states have received more than one hundred reports of medical mistakes from health care facilities. It's obvious that health care facilities don't take medical error reporting seriously.

New York has one of the more active reporting programs that requires hospitals to report errors, and it receives about 15,000 reports a year. The state releases information to the public in the aggregate for each hospital, including the number of reports submitted.

Florida requires hospitals to report errors, such as medical procedures performed on the wrong person, but this information had been kept confidential. Because of growing public pressure for disclosure, a new law approved by the Florida legislature allows state officials to post medical mistakes on the state's Web site, but the name of the health care facility where the mistake was made is omitted, as well as the name of the health professionals involved. While this is a good start, it would be better to know where the error occurred; the publicity provides an incentive for health care providers to improve the safety of the care they render. It's exactly the kind of publicity that hospitals don't want, which is why they are lobbying hard against mandatory reporting of medical errors.

Leonard, whose wife died after she received an epidural from a young resident, requested that the state health department investigate his wife's death. The investigators filed a report saying the hospital violated the state code. Would the hospital have reported the event to the state health department on its own if Leonard had not requested an investigation? Who knows? If hospitals don't have a compelling incentive to report errors, then some of them may not.

The IOM panel recommended that Congress provide funding to states to establish error-reporting systems or adapt their current ones and to collect standardized information, analyze it, and follow up with health care facilities as needed. To date, Congress has not acted. States provide only minuscule funding—only about $20 million is allocated annually in all the states for mandatory reporting of mistakes in a $1.5 trillion health care system. Consequently, states don't have the money to hire staff to collect information, analyze it, or investigate patterns of high volumes of errors. This situation is no different than the chronic underfunding of state medical boards that lack the capacity to respond to concerns of the public.

If mandatory reporting of medical mistakes is to occur, what mistakes should be reported? The National Quality Forum, a nonprofit group made up of influential leaders in health care, identified twenty-seven "never events" that should be reported by all licensed health care facilities. These events include deaths from medical mistakes such as transfusions of the wrong blood type, medication mistakes, and surgeries on the wrong person or body part. A standardized list, developed with the consensus of representatives in health care, makes it easier for states to know which information should be collected. In this way, there will be some uniformity in what the states can report to the public. But the "never events" list is still very new and the states haven't yet adopted them.

Voluntary Reporting

Some forward-looking hospitals and other facilities are initiating voluntary reporting systems. Used for internal quality improvement rather than public reporting, this idea springs from another safety-oriented industry: aviation. The Veterans Health Administration has started a voluntary reporting system and has contracted with the National Aeronautics and Space Administration (NASA) to design and operate it. It's a four-year, $8.2 million agreement that establishes the Patient Safety Reporting System for use in the VA health system nationally.

Why NASA? Because NASA operates the Aviation Safety Reporting System for the Federal Aviation Administration. Pilots, flight attendants, mechanics, air traffic controllers, and others who see or are involved in an aviation situation that could cause harm or compromise safety can submit reports voluntarily and in strict confidence.

In a similar way, NASA will collect and analyze reports of medical mistakes or near misses in VA health care facilities; the information NASA collects will be used to continually improve the safety of health care provided to patients in those facilities. This system has worked for the FAA, and it should work in health care. Just as in the aviation reporting system, any names that identify people or organizations involved will be deleted. With no names attached, employees won't be afraid of reprisal if they report a mistake or a near miss. The voluntary reporting system is a giant leap forward, in that successful strategies for error reduction used in other industries are finally beginning to migrate into health care.

Congress is considering legislation to encourage health care organizations to develop their own voluntary reporting systems by giving legal protection to those who report mistakes. This may be a worthwhile step because voluntary reporting can be a very effective tool to identify where breeding grounds for mistakes are especially nutrient-rich. But it's not good enough if Congressional action leaves out funding for mandatory reporting of errors that result in death or serious injury, as the IOM recommended. Otherwise, we're back to square one, and the public is left in the dark.

Lessons from the aviation sector are relevant here, too. The FAA tracks airplane crash fatalities by airline and makes the information available to the public. While not all travelers use this information when booking flights, the public is likely to feel some comfort knowing that a federal agency is collecting it and publicly reporting it. Airlines can benchmark themselves against one another, another form of checks and balances that does not exist in health care—yet. The public also can report airline safety concerns by contacting the FAA's toll-free number listed in the telephone book.

Would Congress ever think of assuring the safety of passenger air travel by having the FAA use only voluntary reporting of errors and near misses? No, it wouldn't. With as many as 100,000 deaths a year from medical errors, surely the public would want to know that someone is minding the health care store. That's why mandatory reporting of serious errors is essential.

Where Does the Buck Stop?

What happens if a hospital or other health care facility moves at a snail's pace to reduce medical mistakes? Hardly anything. A hospital might be sued by a patient or a patient's family, but malpractice suits don't tend to stimulate system-wide change in a health care facility unless the events are tragic, are reported extensively in the media, harm the hospital's reputation, and remain in the public eye over an extended period of time.

Hospitals with enlightened leaders, who have always been ahead of their peers in ensuring that quality health care is provided, are making error reduction a top priority. But many other hospitals and health care facilities are doing too little.

That's why required reporting of serious medical mistakes, combined with easy public access to this information, would raise the standard. Hospital CEOs and their governing boards would be accountable to the public and would work hard to build a reputation of safety. Public reporting of the most serious errors that result in death and serious injury could be the rising tide that lifts all boats.

Many of us change our behavior when the consequences of the status quo are worse than changing the behavior. People go to work because if they don't have money, the mortgage or rent won't get paid. Automobile owners have the oil checked in their cars because they don't want the car to stall in the middle of the road on the way home from work in rush hour traffic. People stop smoking out of fear of lung cancer and heart attacks.

We all know people—maybe even ourselves—who keep making the same mistakes over and over again. It can be hard to get out of the cycle of mistakes, and the same tendency is true with organizations. Outside forces are needed to boost them into a new orbit, and in the case of the U.S. health care system, an informed American public is potentially the only rocket with enough fuel to get the job done.

America Likes a Winner, but We Pay the Losers

A powerful fuel feeding the health care engine is hindering progress. Errors cost money, and those who make them don't pay for them. Consider the story of a woman who was hospitalized for back surgery, but the surgeon operated on the wrong vertebra. She had to have a second surgery. As she was on the mend, she called her insurance company and told them what had happened and said that they shouldn't reimburse the hospital for the second surgery because it was the result of an error. The insurance company representative had apparently never heard of such a thing and replied, "Well, that's just not how we do it."

In an interesting twist, the woman called the hospital's president and told him the same thing—the hospital shouldn't get paid for the error. She explains, "I received a copy of the bill that was being sent to the insurance company, which is how I knew the hospital billed the insurance company for the second operation. An interesting side note is that the surgeon never billed for the second surgery, but the hospital made sure it got its money."

The patient, who works for a retail clothing business, sees the world very differently than her insurance company or the hospital's president. "If a customer brings back a pair of pants that we sold to him but don't fit right," she says, "we take them back and give him a new pair in the correct size. And for heaven's sake, we don't charge him for *both* pairs of pants."

So errors are costless to hospitals as long as someone pays them for their mistakes—whether it's insurance companies, Medicare, or patients and their families. Many of the people you've met had to pay out-of-pocket for the cost of mistakes and follow-up care to repair the damage. In fact, it would be interesting to find out how hospitals justify bills submitted for the same surgery on the same patient performed within a short period of time. In what other sector of America's economy is this allowed to occur?

Compared with other sectors of the economy, the health care industry's performance is bleak. After the IOM released its report, a government-wide task force prepared a report to President Clinton that compared health care to other industries in the following way: "If performance levels of 99.9 percent—substantially better than those found in the intensive care unit—applied to the airline and banking industries, it would equate to two dangerous landings per day at O'Hare International Airport and 32,000 checks deducted from the wrong account per hour."

No business would survive today in America if it provided as much unsafe service as that provided in the health care system. Yet some health care organizations do survive. This isn't a new phenomenon, as John Ruskin, the nineteenth-century English writer and artist, reminds us, "Yet you pay with equal fee . . . the . . . good and bad workmen upon your body."[2]

Many dedicated people are working hard, though, trying to reduce medical mistakes and give their patients high-quality care. They measure their performance and reduce deaths and injury. This is the best of health care, but the professionals who work so hard at making certain that patients are not harmed are reimbursed no differently than those who provide unsafe and poor-quality care. The conscientious ones are neither recognized nor rewarded for their effort to provide higher-quality care. Meanwhile, the public doesn't know who they are—again because there is no public reporting that separates the wheat from the chaff.

Money Talks

The federal Medicare program doesn't have the resources to provide the level of oversight needed to hold health care facilities accountable for the safety of the care provided to patients. When it does act, it can be very effective. In one instance, federal officials put a hospital in Colorado on probation because of concerns about patient safety, and its reimbursement from Medicare—a staple of a hospital's financial diet—was in jeopardy. The federal government's clout and power of the purse was a powerful motivator for the hospital to change management, hire enough nurses to prevent overworked nurses from making mistakes, and institute other improvements. Surely, the changes were not a pleasant experience for the hospital, especially when its very existence was threatened. But the process worked, and the hospital made improvements.

The hospital CEO told the *Chicago Tribune* that while hospital administrators are dismayed by the public spotlight on a hospital's darkest moments, the accountability has improved care. The CEO also told the *Tribune*, "There are still a lot of other hospitals out there just like we were, I know, because I've seen them. We just were the one that got noticed."[3]

It would be revolutionary to even mention the idea that health care organizations should be paid only if they provide high-quality care. It's even more revolutionary to suggest they shouldn't be paid for providing unsafe, poor-quality care. Yet if errors and substandard care start having a negative impact on health care facilities' bottom lines, preventing them will become a top priority.

part four

Courage to Change
the Things We Can

10 | Making Health Care Safe

A former pilot from New England, who has firsthand experience with medical errors, says, "In health care, they have to do what aviation has done, which is to make it very hard for a pilot to make a mistake." Forward-thinking hospitals *are* trying to reduce the chances that medical mistakes occur, and while their efforts won't eliminate mistakes, they will make it more difficult for errors to happen.

Technology to the Rescue

Apart from information systems to manage their finances and inventories on Web sites that offer general information to the public, most health care facilities have yet to take advantage of all that information technology has to offer. In 1996, the health care industry spent only $543 per worker on information technology compared with $12,666 spent by securities brokers, and it ranked 38 out of 53 industries surveyed for its use of technology.[1]

The good news is that an impressive array of technologies to improve the process of care—as opposed to technology to diagnose or treat patients—is emerging. Here are just a few examples that whet the appetite and hold promise for keeping patients safer.

LIGHT-YEARS BEYOND HANDWRITING

The Brigham and Women's Hospital, a large hospital in Boston that is a teaching affiliate of Harvard Medical School, is an industry leader that is successfully using a computer system to improve the accuracy of medication prescribing. Moving light-years beyond hosting handwriting courses for doctors, as some hospitals are doing, Brigham and Women's started a new system that eliminates prescription orders written by hand. With about 7,000 drug orders coming through the hospital pharmacy every day, mistakes were waiting to happen. Now, a physician orders a prescription drug through a computer, which automatically checks the request against the patient's medical history. If the patient is allergic to the drug or is taking other drugs that might interact with the prescribed medication, the computer raises a red flag.

Other medication errors can be avoided, too. A vexing problem is when patients continue to receive a medication after the doctor has ordered it to be discontinued. The electronic system has "stop-dates" that make it impossible for the hospital staff to forget that a patient is still being administered a certain medication. If the physician stops prescribing a medication, the computer prevents a nurse from dispensing the drug by sending a signal to the medicine cabinet on the hospital ward.

Medication errors at Brigham and Women's have decreased 55 percent since the new system was instituted. Fewer drugs are being ordered at dosages that exceed the recommended maximum. The new system is also helping doctors improve how they prescribe. Patients undergoing certain cancer treatment can suffer nausea, and now, more patients are receiving anti-nausea medications. In fact, the increase was dramatic. Previously, doctors followed appropriate prescribing only 6 percent of the time. Now, it's 75 percent. This means that a lot more people are more comfortable while undergoing treatment.

Yet even with answers to medical mistakes within reach, more than 95 percent of hospitals still use old-fashioned pen and paper.

tes on patients, and databases with information on diseases that
n help them make quicker and more accurate diagnoses. Slowly
t surely, technology is coming to the patient's bedside. In the
ure, medical students won't be carrying index cards and scraps
paper in their pockets to remember important information. In
t, their faculty, many of whom are part of the generation that
ln't have personal computers at home, are learning from their
dical students and residents about how technology can improve
care they provide to their patients.

Major corporations are stepping up to the plate to push the
alth care system into the technology age. General Motors, the
gest private payer of health care costs in the country, is spon-
ing the distribution of handheld units to about 5,000 physicians
o treat GM employees. Doctors who use the handheld units will
able to prescribe medications and access patients' health care
ords, reference materials, and other key information electroni-
ly.

MMY MEDICINE

uld commercial airlines or federal regulators allow pilots to
rn to fly a plane for the first time on a flight across the Atlantic
ean with 369 passengers on board? Of course not. Pilots train
flight simulators and are taught how to respond to crises. The
velopment of flight simulators after World War II represented a
w way to train pilots to fly increasingly sophisticated aircraft and
uce pilot error. If aviation was to evolve from military use to
nmercial use by the traveling public, simulators were—and still
—an essential form of training.

Is there an alternative to doctors "learning by doing" on living
ients—sometimes in cases of life and death? Why not use sim-
tors to train doctors? Thanks to the emergence of "dummy
dicine," some doctors are starting to train on "dummies," or
ulated patients made of computer chips, wires, and plastic.

Only 2 to 5 percent of hospitals have invested th
to purchase such a computer system and to teac
and pharmacists to make it work. Brigham and
tal's initial investment was almost $2 million ar
are about $500,000 annually. But savings acc
appropriate uses of drugs, fewer mistakes, and e
dant lab tests have yielded a ten- to twentyfold
tial investment.

Even the best of computerized systems are nc
create new opportunities for error. In another
computerized prescription ordering, a physician
it has reduced mistakes from illegible handwritin
problems. "I was at the computer ordering a pr
eighty-year-old patient of mine and, by mistake
clicked on the name of the drug right above the c
prescribe. The drugs on the "pick" list on the com
listed in alphabetical order, and both drugs cor
dosages. Fortunately, the patient was astute and cal
got home and said she had the wrong drug."

The same doctor goes on to say, "Even with th
ordering, I still have to rely on memory. I wantec
medication for a patient I have known for a while
to remember that he became dizzy when taking it. 1
on our system to flag things like that. So if I didn't
tutional memory about this patient, he could have b
a medication he shouldn't have." The lesson learn
new systems for prescribing medications are tools th
improvements, but they are not foolproof.

WIRED DOCTORS ARE NO LONGER WEIRD

The up-and-coming generation of doctors is embra
ogy that can reduce errors. Medical students now
handheld computers that provide information on c

Pioneered at the VA/Stanford Medical Center in Palo Alto, California, dummies can be programmed as a healthy teenager or a frail old man. A dummy can have a heart attack or an allergic reaction to medicine. The severity and responsiveness to treatment can be programmed, and the dummy responds as a real live human being would respond to more than seventy different medications.

In the "operating room," doctors and nurses can participate in simulated surgeries. The "patient" might be undergoing routine knee surgery that turns nearly lethal as the "patient's" heart rate accelerates sharply and blood pressure drops precipitously. Dummies are programmed to simulate movements such as breathing and heart function and can have different symptoms and respond differently, depending on the surgical team's actions. The procedures can be videotaped so the team can watch and assess how well they did. Dummies are currently being used for medical education and training around the world, and "dummy medicine" will eventually become a common way for doctors and nurses to learn to perform new techniques or use new technology.

Of course, just because someone is trained on a simulator doesn't mean he or she will be skilled in caring for a living human being. Nonetheless, "dummy medicine" represents an important technological tool for training new doctors and providing continuing education for experienced doctors. The good news is that training on simulators is becoming more common, although it's still limited. Surgeons can now use simulators to learn how to do some types of orthopedic and sinus surgery. This is a good start, but health care has a long way to go before it catches up to other industries that use simulators to improve the quality of what they do.

FROM SUPERMARKET TO SURGICAL SUITE

It has been said that wise people learn from their mistakes, and those who don't are bound to repeat them. The Department of Veterans Affairs established its National Center for Patient Safety in

1998 as an umbrella for all its initiatives to improve safety, including the voluntary reporting system described earlier. The VA wants to learn from its mistakes and try to prevent them. In fact, in 2001, the Center won a prestigious award for Innovation in American Government, bestowed annually by the Kennedy School of Government at Harvard University.

Among its many initiatives, the VA is implementing bar-code technology to reduce mistakes. Bar codes, those little patterns of thin and thick lines printed on virtually everything we buy these days, are coming to health care. All VA facilities are now required to use bar-code technology in hospital operating rooms to make sure patients receive the blood product meant for them. In a pilot test at the Topeka, Kansas, VA medical center, the use of bar codes reduced medication mistakes by almost 70 percent. This shouldn't be a surprise, since nearly every company that has used bar codes to track products finds that this simple and very inexpensive technology dramatically cuts mistakes.

Here is how it works. A nurse scans the bar code on the container of medication or blood product and then scans the bar code on the patient's wristband to make sure that the right drug is being given to the right patient. This technology is an added check to the standard verification, when two people visually check the patient's identity to be sure it matches the information on the blood product. Bar codes will eventually be universal. The U.S. Food and Drug Administration intends to require bar codes on every drug that is dispensed. While hospital and pharmaceutical companies express support for bar coding, they say it will take years to implement. The public's growing concern over medical errors and what the industry is doing (or not doing) to curtail them can speed up that timetable.

IT TAKES A VILLAGE

Technology can't prevent all the breakdowns that result in harm to patients. More often than not, better communication is needed among and within the different tribes in health care that are taking care of the same patient. Just outside Washington, D.C., a 217-bed community hospital started using a team approach in 1996 to care for patients in its intensive care unit. According to a *USA Today* account, the team includes a doctor who is a specialist in intensive care medicine, the chief ICU nurse, a pharmacist, a social worker, a nutritionist, a respiratory therapist, and a chaplain. The team visits each patient and discusses as a group the best course of action for the patient. So instead of one doctor saying one thing to a patient and another saying something different, the team conveys a consistent message to the patient and the family. The hospital found that fewer mistakes and complications have occurred with this team approach. It costs more in direct costs for staffing, but with fewer mishaps, patients spend less time in the high-cost intensive care unit, which cuts down on human misery and saves money overall.[2]

Pressure Soars

What will it take to have hospitals and other health care facilities embrace technology and other improvements for the sake of their patients' safety? The Leapfrog Group is finding out. The Business Roundtable, an association of chief executive officers of leading corporations, spearheaded the establishment of the Leapfrog Group, a consortium of one hundred and twenty public and private organizations including Fortune 500 companies such as GM, Boeing, Kodak, IBM, Motorola, Northwest Airlines, and others. Together, they pay for the health care benefits of more than 33 million Americans, and along with their employees, spend more than $52 billion on health care each year.

Helping to fuel the work of the Leapfrog Group was an internal report at GM that estimated that four hundred and eighty-eight GM employees, retirees, and their family members die from medical mistakes each year—a number that hit too close to home. The idea behind the Leapfrog Group is to have those who pay the health care bills in America use their clout to pressure health care organizations to deliver quality care. After all, if automakers demand excellence from their suppliers of steel and auto parts, for example, why shouldn't they require excellence in the quality of health care provided to their employees who make the cars we drive?

The goal of the group is to give patient safety a giant "leap" forward. As Bruce Bradley, a GM executive, put it, "The current health care environment is untenable. There's just too much waste in the system—and we're not talking about tongue depressors here. We're talking about injuries, disabilities, and lost lives from medical mistakes."[3]

So how can businesses and other big payers of America's health care bill encourage more hospitals to invest in lifesaving technology of the kind that Brigham and Women's hospital is using? The Leapfrog Group is trying, and here's an example of how market clout works.

Boeing Corporation and the International Association of Machinists and Aerospace Workers (IAM) have a large presence in the Pacific Northwest. Representatives of both groups met individually with each of the CEOs of the twenty-six hospitals in the area. In one of the meetings, a union member asked the hospital CEO to invest in computerized prescription technology because someone he knew had suffered the effects of a medication error. The hospital CEO replied that its capital investment budget couldn't handle another expenditure. Yet a company representative who had done his homework pointed out that the hospital's capital expenditure budget included spending to improve some of the aesthetic aspects of the hospital. The hospital CEO said he would look into their request. The hospital has since made a commitment to establish computerized prescribing by 2004—along with the other twenty-five hospitals in the area.

The IAM and companies including Boeing, Raytheon, and Bombardier are using the same strategy to leverage their market muscle in Wichita, Kansas, which is home to 25,000 IAM-represented employees and 50,000 other employees. Their work will affect not just the employees but the entire community. IAM's Steve Sleigh says, "Perhaps it is not surprising that an industry like aerospace, where quality production is so critical, or that a union like the IAM with its highly skilled membership, would take the lead in creating value in this manner."[4]

The Leapfrog Group is identifying those hospitals that are investing in computerized ordering of prescriptions, and the information can be found by logging on to www.leapfroggroup.org and clicking on "hospital survey results." Listed there are the names of hospitals that have agreed to provide information on whether they have already implemented new systems or are planning to do so and whether they are willing to report to their communities their progress in reducing medication errors.

These results, which come from a survey that hospitals completed voluntarily, provide some indication of a hospital's commitment to reduce medication errors. There's no tracking or measuring of medication errors, at least not yet. This could be the next step after the infrastructure is in place.

Most of the Leapfrog information is for hospitals in eighteen regions of the United States, in addition to some hospitals outside these regions that have also submitted information. With about 5,000 hospitals in the country, there's still a long way to go. Legislation had been introduced in Congress to help provide financial support for rural and inner-city hospitals to help them defray the cost of this technology, but it stalled, and federal budget constraints probably mean that no help is likely to be forthcoming in the foreseeable future.

PASS THE KETCHUP, BUT NO MEDICAL MISTAKES, PLEASE

The big ketchup maker, H.J. Heinz, is one of at least thirty large and small companies in Pittsburgh that are paying close attention to medical mistakes occurring in the area's hospitals. Along with Alcoa and other employers in Pittsburgh, the companies are testing the mettle of health care providers to see if they can eliminate medication errors and other mistakes.

In Pittsburgh, the Regional Health Care Initiative was created in 1997 with the aim of having employers contract only with those hospitals and doctors that commit to reducing errors and improving the overall quality of care. These Pittsburgh companies want health care leaders to learn how to do a complete "makeover" of the way they provide health care. In many ways, this is little different from the makeover that many Pittsburgh companies went through in the 1980s and 1990s to produce a higher-quality product with fewer defects and reduce costs so they could survive the competition from overseas producers. Paul O'Neill, the former Chairman and CEO of Alcoa, and former Treasury Secretary in the Bush Administration, has been a driving force behind Pittsburgh's leading-edge effort. He's convinced that health care organizations can learn from the quality management principles that were pioneered at Toyota and refined at Alcoa. It's too soon to tell the outcome, but at least lessons learned from other sectors of the economy are gradually being applied to health care.

Meanwhile, in New York, four large companies—IBM, PepsiCo, Verizon Communications, and Xerox—are offering hospitals $2 million in incentive payments if they make health care safer. The cash bonuses will start flowing to hospitals when they start using computerized systems to prevent medication mistakes and institute other steps to prevent errors. Hospitals are eligible to receive a 4 percent bonus based on the amount of the care they provide to patients who are employees or retirees of the four companies and insured by Empire Blue Cross and Blue Shield. These four companies provide coverage to more than 100,000 employees and their families in the New York area. About one hundred and fifty hospitals are eligible for the incentive payments, but fewer than ten are using computerized systems to order medications.

Light-Years to Go

So where do things stand since the December 1999 IOM report on national estimates of deaths from medical errors? Even with all of the well-intended efforts noted above, and many more that are being spearheaded by dedicated people in health care facilities around the country, they are voluntary, ad hoc, and sporadic. The pace of improvement is nowhere near what should be expected when as many as 100,000 people die every year. This sad state of affairs prompted the *Washington Post*, in December 2002, to refer to the inaction as "A Medical Enron" that is indicative of "the arrogance of the medical priesthood."

No person, organization, public or private, has the responsibility and authority to ensure that medical errors in the U.S. health care system are drastically reduced—and no one is accountable. This means that the health care industry and the medical profession don't take preventable deaths and injuries from medical errors seriously. And that's where things stand as the United States enters the twenty-first century and spends $1.5 trillion a year on health care.

11 | Honesty, Healing, and Hope

Dear Doctor:

I really don't know why I am writing this. For some reason I feel the need to. I don't hate you. You were a nice man when I met you and I'm sure you're a nice man now. My life was torn apart when my son died and can never fully be put back together again. Michael was my first born, my only child, he was my whole life. Through carelessness he was taken away forever. I've spent many nights and awakened many mornings wondering if I should go to be with my son. I wonder if I'll ever stop feeling this way.

I wonder often if you were leaving for vacation or had a dinner engagement that you didn't want to miss, if this is why Michael wasn't checked further. Were you too busy? I'm sure you're a good doctor. But the saying is, 'a baker eats his mistakes, a doctor buries his.' The mistakes made by this group of doctors have destroyed many lives.

You asked me once if I was going to sue you. I didn't know. I needed answers and had no one to ask. I had to know that it wasn't my mistake.

I know your life isn't going to be disrupted by my tragedy, and I want your children to always feel proud that their daddy

*is a good doctor. But I only pray that every mother who brings
her child to you is a reminder that that child is a piece of her
heart, and you think of my son, Michael Louis, and my heart.*
    Sincerely,
    Ilene

Like many other parents, spouses, children, siblings, and
friends whose hearts are broken in the aftermath of a medical mistake, Ilene wanted to know why her son died and whether she was
a good mother and did all she possibly could to save his life. Her
motivation to write this letter to the doctor who performed the
tonsillectomy and examined the boy afterward is the same as any
mother would have whose child died a preventable death. She
needed to know the answers so she could begin to heal from the
tragedy.

In the heat of the debate over medical errors, hospitals and doctors say they can't disclose medical mistakes because of advice
from lawyers, fear of litigation, and the culture of silence. But disclosure of errors is so important to the people who matter most—
as you'll hear in the words of those who know best.

All of the people and families who have been touched by medical mistakes have one thing in common. They want an acknowledgment that a terrible tragedy has occurred, they want to be told
the truth so they can understand what happened, and they want
someone to "own up" to the fact that a mistake was made. With a
heartfelt, "I'm sorry, we made a mistake," healing can begin not
just for the patients and their families, but also the doctors, nurses,
and others involved. Without honesty, there is no healing. Without healing, there is little hope that doctors and nurses, patients
and families, and hospitals will work together to prevent future
mistakes.

The Silence Is Deafening

In the aftermath of Justin's death from an infection that was undiagnosed, the nineteen-year-old's parents sued the hospital for one simple reason: they wanted the truth. "The hospital wouldn't tell us anything. Neither would the doctor." The wall of silence leaves a family full of understandable anger and rage.

The silence and denial manifest themselves in different human behaviors. Some physicians literally run away and hide. While Susan was in the emergency room waiting for repair surgery to stop the deadly infection raging through her body, the physician who had performed the original laparoscopic procedure that punctured her colon and then ignored the obvious symptoms of infection was just down the hall. That doctor never came to reassure the frightened and extremely ill patient that everything possible was being done to restore her health.

Patients want their doctors to say, "I am so sorry. We'll work to fix this, and if I can't do it, or if you don't want me to, I'll help you find someone who can." A humane response mitigates the feeling of abandonment that compounds the fear when one's life is in grave danger.

When running away isn't an option, it's not hard for doctors and hospitals to ignore a family's questions. Ockie's daughter, Rebecca, describes how the hospital and staff evaded the family. "They didn't answer our questions. The hospital officials really need some insight—if this were your loved one, wouldn't you want answers? If that institution would have called us and said 'This is what happened, we are so very sorry, what can we do to help your family?' they would never have had to deal with a lawsuit from us," explained Rebecca. "We need healing. Treating people like human beings helps families heal."

Legal action may be the only way for some patients and families to get the answers they need about why their loved one died or was injured. And after exhausting all other measures, it may be the last resort to hold someone accountable for a preventable death or injury. But for those who do "win," sometimes the victory can be hollow. It can never bring back the life that once was.

"When did I get an attorney? When the doctors wouldn't apologize to an eight-year old girl," says Leila whose daughter, Elizabeth, had cancer that was left undiagnosed for three months. "And I grew up not liking lawyers. But the doctors didn't believe Elizabeth, and they needed to apologize. I can live with the mistake, but I can't live with the fact that they wouldn't apologize to my daughter, who is permanently disabled. I will go to my grave not understanding it."

It's not hard to understand why people and their families have such anger when they believe they are being lied to. Sandy, whose dad, Claudie, died from a mistake that occurred when his prescription for heparin was refilled incorrectly, describes it plain and simple. She says, "Just think if my neighbor is driving down the road in front of my house, and I'm looking out my window and see him hit my dog, who was running across the street. If he gets out of his car and picks up my dog and brings him up to the house, truly sad and upset for what happened, how can I be mad at him? I would try to make him feel not so bad for something he certainly didn't intend to do. But if he kept on driving and later comes up to the house, lies to me, and says he didn't do it, and yet I saw him do it, you can imagine how mad that would make me feel."

A Policy of Honesty

Conscientious doctors understand the value of honesty, not only with themselves as professionals dedicated to the highest possible standards but also with their patients. One doctor described how a mistake was handled honestly with a grieving family. "The hospital risk manager asked me to review the care provided to an elderly woman who had had hip surgery. She was discharged home, and after several days, her hip wound burst open, and pus was coming out, a sign of a deep wound infection from which she eventually died. The family was concerned that the care was mismanaged and may have resulted in her death.

"I looked at the record, which showed that the nurses had documented that the patient had had a fever right before she was discharged from the hospital, a sign of possible infection. But it was not acted on. The physician was not notified, nor did he pick up on it. So there was some warning that something was going on. I reviewed the chart and concluded that the family did have a legitimate concern.

"A meeting was called with the family and in attendance were the hospital risk manager, the hospital medical director (who is also an anesthesiologist), the orthopedic surgeon, and myself. One of the woman's daughters was a nurse case manager who worked at a nearby hospital. The surgeon and anesthesiologist talked about the many reasons that people fare poorly after surgery and how these kinds of complications can occur. They seemed intent on saying they were not to blame, which is what usually happens. On some level, it sweeps things under the carpet. Clearly becoming frustrated, the family responded to the excuses and explanations by asking more questions. One daughter demanded to know why a whole series of things had happened.

"At this point I said to the family, 'I want you to know that we are very, very sorry that your wife and mother died. We feel for your loss. We will do our best to make sure that nothing like this happens again.' The two daughters burst into tears. The family needed the doctors and the hospital to acknowledge that something terrible had happened to the wife and mother they loved. They needed to know that we were profoundly sorry for what had happened, and we would do our very best to prevent it from happening to anyone else. The change in the atmosphere in the room after my comments was palpable. The husband also got teary, and they actually thanked me as they left.

"After the meeting, I worked with the nurses in the unit and we changed the procedure to ensure there was clear documentation when a vital sign is abnormal and that it is brought to the physician's attention."

Some patients and families want more than "I'm sorry." They want doctors and hospitals to acknowledge not just the fact that a mistake occurred, but that *they* made a mistake. To hear someone say "The buck stops here" helps them make sense of the tragedy they're going through.

Another doctor describes how the "buck" stopped with her while caring for a patient. "An error occurred with a patient of mine—he wasn't harmed but it was a bad experience. After he went home, I wrote a letter expressing my apology to him for the mistake. I outlined the corrective steps that had been taken to prevent another patient from suffering from the same flaws in the system.

"I didn't tell the hospital or the risk management department about my letter to the patient. If I had, they wouldn't have let me send it because I actually admitted to the patient that a mistake occurred. And the hospital is so paranoid and doesn't want to be sued. So it never wants to acknowledge that a mistake has been made. But telling the truth is the only ethical thing to do. As his physician, I had an obligation to tell him what happened, why it happened, and what is being done to prevent it from happening again."

The Joint Commission on the Accreditation of Healthcare Organizations recognizes the value of disclosure and now requires hospitals, as part of the hospital accreditation process, to disclose medical mistakes to patients and families. Though certainly an important step in the right direction, a new requirement doesn't mean that errors will suddenly be disclosed, in part because the consequences of nondisclosure are not severe enough for hospitals to take the well-intended requirement seriously.

How often are medical errors disclosed and apologies rendered? In a survey led by researchers at the Harvard School of Public Health, doctors and members of the public were asked about their experiences with medical mistakes.[1] The survey respondents who reported a firsthand experience with a medical mistake were then asked whether the health care professionals involved in the mistake disclosed the error or apologized to them. About a third of both groups answered in the affirmative, saying the error was disclosed or apologies were rendered.

Some patients and families express appreciation when a medical mistake is disclosed. Here's what Diana says of her experience in the hospital that was more safety conscious than the one that didn't even have enough staff to take care of her. "What impressed me most was the way potentially adverse circumstances were handled. Shortly after surgery, I had a reaction to the anesthesia that required monitoring for several days. As soon as I regained consciousness, I was apprised of the circumstances by a team of doctors and nurses from cardiology, orthopedics, and pain management. Their honesty, openness, and constant communication with me and each other put me at ease and gave me great confidence in their skill and good judgment. How different from my earlier experience!"

The Economics of Honesty

Though some doctors are honest with their patients and tell them the truth, the coverup of medical mistakes is the status quo in health care today. For many hospital administrators and doctors, and the lawyers who advise them to keep quiet, the status quo makes sound economic sense. Or does it? Many patients and families say they would not sue if they were told the truth. The authors of a study published in the journal *Archives of Internal Medicine* reported that when medical mistakes are covered up, the risk of litigation almost doubles.[2]

Honesty can be a good policy against lawsuits, as was the case with Claudie, the retired factory foreman from Kentucky. After Claudie died of a blood clot in his lung because of a medication error, the VA hospital that treated him reviewed the events surrounding his care. About three weeks after he died, a lawyer and a nurse from the VA drove an hour and a half to the family's home and asked some questions about Claudie's prescription medicines and the care he received. They left and came back a few weeks later, and what they said surprised Claudie's family. Sandy recalls the lawyer and the nurse from the VA saying, "You were right, we were the ones responsible for your dad's death." They admitted that the hospital pharmacy made a mistake when the staff refilled her dad's prescription for heparin at 10 percent of the dose he should have received to prevent blood clots. Sandy suspected this all along because she had in her possession the empty bottles of medicine that didn't match what was written on the prescription. "They apologized and they cried along with us," Sandy remembers. "It was as if God had come down and taken all this weight off my shoulders. I can't tell you the healing that happens when the truth comes out. It takes away the guilt I felt because I was giving Dad his medicine and I was beating myself up over it."

The VA staff invited Claudie's family to come to the hospital to see the changes made in the pharmacy to prevent medication mistakes from happening to other patients. Procedures had been revamped, and staffing changes in the pharmacy permitted more pharmacists to be on duty during peak hours throughout the day.

Honesty brings more than healing. It builds trust. After her father died, some time passed, and Sandy's mother needed to be admitted to the hospital. She went to the University of Kentucky, which is adjacent to the VA medical center. Sandy asked a VA doctor to come and take a look at her mother. "How many people who lose a dad at someone's hands would then ask the same people to take care of their mother?" she asks.

Sandy's experience is not unique. Other patients at the Lexington VA Medical Center benefit because it has had a policy of disclosure of medical mistakes since 1987. The policy is based on an understanding that medical mistakes are going to occur, patients and families want full disclosure, and they should be offered compensation. Patients and families are not viewed as adversaries and instead are elevated to a status that accords them special attention. Mistakes are disclosed even when the patients or family members are unaware that they occurred.

The medical center's total malpractice payments are on the low end compared with a large group of similar VA facilities. Less money is spent on lawyers and expert witnesses by avoiding long and expensive lawsuits. For its forthrightness about its mistakes, the hospital has achieved national and international recognition. In fact, the medical center invites the media to interview patients and families who have borne the effects of mistakes.

Dr. Steven Kraman, the chief of staff at the medical center who has led this noble effort, says, "Health care organizations should deal with their inevitable mistakes in the same manner as honest people do when erring in their private lives: apologize, compensate fairly, and try to avoid making the same mistake again."[3]

Diana, the former Air Force intelligence officer, would agree. As she said in testimony before the U.S. Congress, "We've got to get beyond an 'us' versus 'them' mentality, with doctors and hospitals covering up their mistakes and refusing to acknowledge them. Unless they are willing and able to admit their mistakes, learn from them, and promptly correct them, we will widen the chasm of distrust between 'us' and 'them.'" The Lexington VA Medical Center has shown a way to narrow that chasm and build the trust between the people who come to them for healing and those who care for them. It also shows that while the threat of being sued is a serious impediment to acknowledging medical mistakes, it is possible to learn how to create a culture that is accountable and learns from its mistakes.

Healing the Healers

Patients and families are not the only ones that need answers and healing when a medical mistake occurs. A mother whose child died from a medical mistake astutely acknowledges that conscientious doctors and nurses feel tremendous guilt and profound sadness when they are involved in a medical mistake that causes harm. She says, "There is no support for those who make errors. There is no training in medical schools on how to handle it." If doctors have been taught in medical school to bury their mistakes, and if the culture where they work enforces this teaching, they may have never seen another doctor say the words that disclose mistakes and offer apologies to a family. And doctors learn by watching their peers.

Elizabeth's mother, Leila, echoes the same observation. Using her daughter's story as a learning opportunity for future doctors, she participated in a course in the medical school near where she lives. "I want to see physicians and nurses heal," and her daughter understands this, too. She recalls how Elizabeth was sitting on the front porch one day and said, "I feel sorry for those doctors. You have to know they must feel bad about what happened." Her mom goes on to say, "The doctors missed the chance to hear Elizabeth say, 'I know you didn't mean to hurt me. I forgive you.' There is so much richness in these words, but the doctors missed it. And they know deep down they screwed up, and it must be so painful."

Calls for Compassion

In July 1996, Congress passed the Aviation Disaster Family Assistance Act in response to the pleas of relatives of victims of airplane crashes. The law requires airlines to offer assistance to family members in the aftermath of a crash—for example, making hotel rooms and food available and offering crisis counseling to grieving families.

Hospitals don't provide that support, as Lewis's mother, Helen, described so poignantly in her journal. "My husband and a nurse supervisor clear our belongings out of his hospital room with his body lying on the bed. My husband and daughter get the car and drive back to the motel. I am not ready to leave my child and try to stay and sit in the hall, still clutching the clean pillow I had been planning to put on his bed that morning. The ward resumes its normal activity and I realize it is futile to stay. The pastor says he will have security drive me back to the motel. We go downstairs and the pastor leaves. I am driven back to the motel in a police car by two security guards talking about paint. It's the last we hear from any of the hospital's 'support services.'" Helen continues, "In our experience, all contact with the family was left up to the physician. This is a heavy burden to impose on the doctor. It is also completely inadequate to meet the needs of a family that has just suffered a shocking tragedy. Hospitals need to have a support system in place, not just for medical error victims but for families of any patient who dies in the hospital. I will never forget the way we were simply turned out into the street. The only call we ever got from the hospital was asking if we would donate our son's eyes. In the best of worlds, hospitals would cooperate with, perhaps even sponsor, advocacy groups assisting victims of medical mistakes. Hospitals would acknowledge the mistake and call patient advocates to come to the family's aid as soon as the mistake was known."

The insensitivity to a patient's ordeal can be striking. Dick is a retired store manager whose colon was punctured during a colonoscopy. He subsequently developed a raging infection that very nearly killed him. Several months afterward, while Dick was still recovering, he received several bills from the doctor who did the colonoscopy, along with the usual form letter asking, "How are we doing?" "Would you recommend us?" Dick's wife, Jeanne, said, "Having been brought up a lady, I just tore it up." She had almost lost her lifelong companion, an experience no wife ever wants to go through, and the doctor never apologized, expressed his regret at what happened, or showed any sensitivity to their ordeal.

Health care organizations will provide support to patients and families who are living in the aftermath of a medical mistake only when they can admit that they made a mistake. If they don't admit a mistake was made, they can't empathize with the people who live with the consequences. Nor will they realize the obligation they have to offer patients and families the support they need to go on living.

A mother writes, "For a bereaved parent, the idea that you will survive while your child does not is the most awful concept there is. You pray for death, or at least madness. It doesn't come, of course. There are only two things that bring any surcease. One is simply the mind's inability to take in this sort of perversion of the natural order. You carry on because you don't believe it. The second is the support of other people. People—sometimes people you have never even met—are just astonishing in their willingness to be there."

Will doctors, nurses, and hospital staff be there for other mothers and fathers, sons and daughters, husbands and wives? Unfortunately, we think it will take a long time before they muster the courage to support patients and families who suffer harm in the aftermath of a medical mistake. But in the interim, a cadre of compassionate people is stepping forward and showing us all how to do so.

Works of Mercy

Those who have experienced medical mistakes themselves have begun to offer comfort, support, and advice to others who are just discovering the depths of agony and despair that accompany a medical error. Dying or being injured while receiving medical care—and being turned away and ignored when it happens—is devastating.

Throughout our lives we are taught that doctors help us heal, not make us sick. We expect that we won't be abandoned when we need them most. We expect that hospitals are one of the safest places in the world. We expect that doctors and nurses will act in an ethical manner. When these expectations are not met, and when patients and families are abandoned, lied to, and treated in an unethical manner, emotions run deep and across the gamut of anger, rage, vulnerability, fear, sadness. Victims feel betrayed by the very people who they thought would help them. Navigating these uncharted waters is a solitary journey, made ever more difficult by the fact that one is wounded physically, emotionally, and financially.

Jennifer is an advocate who started a grassroots group for victims of medical mistakes. Jennifer's mother died from mistakes and substandard care, and Jennifer and other families who had experienced mistakes gathered together in February of 1996 to discuss medical errors. The people who participated began to ask questions and wanted to learn more about why their loved one died and why. They began to question why the hospital or the state medical board took no action when the care provided to their loved ones or themselves resulted in harm.

This was the beginning of PULSE (Persons United Limiting Substandards and Errors in Health Care) of Colorado in 1996, whose goal is to help the public become aware of potential adversities in the health care system and knowledgeable about which are due to medical errors and which are not. Jennifer tries to teach others how to recognize the difference. Having served on the board of a local community health center, she understands both sides— as a daughter of a loved one who died and as one involved in the governance of a health care facility.

In her work with PULSE, Jennifer was contacted by several concerned families who had experiences with medical mistakes that all involved the same doctor. An inveterate networker, she put them in touch with each other and advised them how to file complaints with the state medical board. When multiple and similar complaints were filed that were hard for the medical board to ignore, the tactic worked. The doctor voluntarily retired.

In another instance, Jennifer helped a woman who was grieving after she lost her child to substandard care and was so afraid of having another child, lest she lose that one, too. Jennifer put her in touch with another woman who also lost a child due to a medical mistake and who went on to have several more children. The first mother gained confidence from her friendship with another grieving mom and went on to have a healthy, happy child.

Financially strapped families also have benefited from the good works of PULSE. "We've had a couple of fundraisers for families—pizza parties, spaghetti dinners, yard and bake sales," says Jennifer. "We do the legwork and get the event organized, but have the family, church, or fraternal organization take care of the money. We held one event to raise money so a family could pay the burial expenses for their son. It's not just about the money," she says. "It's a way for us to show people that somebody cares."

Why does Jennifer volunteer her time to do this work? She explains, "My mother has been gone for seven years, yet at times it still hurts as if it were yesterday that I had to say goodbye. There is some healing for me when I see others move forward after getting the support and answers they need to survive their loss. If I can do a small part in changing the system that lets this happen, then I have done something worthy in this world."

PULSE has grown into a grassroots network with chapters in several states. Thousands of miles away, Ilene, Michael's mom, started a state chapter of PULSE in New York. She saw a story on a local television station about a bill pending in the New York state legislature that would have made background information on physicians licensed to practice in New York available to the public. The reporter noted that the bill was not likely to pass, a situation that outraged Ilene. She helped to spearhead a grassroots effort to make sure that if not this bill, then another would eventually make it into law. On a mission to give the public better information and make the health care system more accountable to those who matter most—the patients, Ilene lobbied hospital executives, politicians, doctors, nurses, and people who know firsthand the impact of medical mistakes.

On October 6, 2000, when George Pataki, the Governor of New York, signed into law the bill making information about doctors licensed to practice in the state publicly accessible (www.nydoctorprofile.com), Ilene was invited to be present. The law can't bring Ilene's son, Michael, back. But it is a step toward more disclosure, honesty, and accountability in health care—which is the only way that no other family will have to endure unspeakable loss.

In addition to her advocacy, Ilene helps support victims of medical mistakes. Ilene befriended a woman whose husband died after egregious errors. To this day, ten years later, the woman is still hurting and consumed with anger about her husband's unnecessary death. Ilene says, "She needed to safely share her anger about the fact that the system killed her husband. It's a story she couldn't share for ten years because no one could understand. Who are you going to talk to when you think your loved one was harmed in the health care system? It's not something you talk about at the dinner table with friends. . . . But now I see my friend being transformed as she gets past the anger—which is a sign that there is a hurting person inside. And I like her so much as a person. We can do so much good by listening and being a friend."

The grassroots network of patient safety advocates also has become a haven for health care professionals—doctors, nurses, pharmacists, and administrators—who contact them to share their worries, fears, grief, and frustrations. Linked mostly by phone and the Internet, these virtual networks are a safe haven where professional caregivers can talk about safety concerns, which many cannot do in the unsupportive health facilities where they work. Calls come in from people in tears because they almost harmed someone because of the careless systems in which they work.

The task of providing comfort to victims of medical mistakes—both the patients and families, as well as the professional caregivers—has been left in the hands of those who have suffered themselves. It is they who understand and who volunteer to help those harmed by the health care system, tend to their wounds, and help them heal.

The Need for a New Covenant

Will people who have suffered from medical mistakes ever find comfort and support in the place where they were harmed? Will health care organizations do good when bad things happen? It depends on whether they rethink their covenant with the patients they are supposed to serve.

We learned about a small group of doctors in rural northern Michigan who get up before dawn to meet regularly before their full day of work to discuss ways they can better understand patients' needs—beyond those that medicine, as we know it, endeavors to meet. They gather together to try to be better doctors. At one of their regular meetings, the doctors invited a woman in her forties who was dying from cancer to talk with them—she was still able to come even in the advanced stages of cancer. They asked her, "What has been most helpful from the medical community during this difficult year?" She candidly replied, "Nothing. The only reason I'm still alive is my family and friends." The silence was deafening. The professionals had missed seeing the things that were most important to her. She died about two weeks later, in the evening, having attended her son's hockey game that morning.

This woman's professional caregivers had seen the illness and had done their best to treat it. But they didn't see the person behind the illness, or understand the events in her life that sustained it in ways that medicine cannot. All good doctors know that patients are the best teachers. Yet, as some of the best doctors in the country concede, they themselves are not the best listeners. By listening to people who have experienced a preventable death or injury in the health system, the prospects for learning, improving, and even having a change of heart are enormous.

Those who have been harmed say they want a "voice," but what are they really saying? Beyond the label given to them as "patient" or "family member," they want to be recognized for the person who they are. They want others to know that the life that was lost to error—their beloved son or daughter, mother or father, husband or wife—was someone whose life had great meaning but has been senselessly taken away. Who of us would not want a voice?

Hospital CEOs Set the Tone

How many hospital CEOs and chiefs of medicine meet with patients and families who have borne the consequence of medical error? How often do they render their sincere regret, and commit themselves to make the health care they provide as safe as it can be? Far too few.

A woman we met described how she tried to make an appointment to meet with the CEO of the health care organization where her mother died from a medical mistake. She says it took months to get an appointment, and when she did, she traveled several hours to meet the CEO in his office. She recalls her meeting with him this way, "When I arrived, I was ushered into the corporate conference room, and he had an entire entourage with him, which didn't lend itself to an intimate discussion of the very personal issues I wanted to discuss. I had my questions for him about the circumstances that allowed my mother's death to occur and asked specifically about the various aspects of the system to ensure that events like my mother's death didn't happen again. His rote response to each question was, 'I don't know, I'll have to check into that and get back to you.' After a short while, he looked at his watch and said he had only a few minutes because he had to take his daughter to the beach. I never heard from the man again."

Another missed opportunity for healing—and a recommitment to the safety of patients. Imagine the CEO of an airline saying the same thing to the daughter of a woman who died in a plane crash.

Contrast this approach to how a hospital in Tokyo responded to a medical mistake that was covered up. The *Daily Yomiuri*, a Tokyo newspaper, reported that a twelve-year-old patient died as a result of medical errors committed during a heart operation.[4] To take responsibility for the fatality, the director of the Heart Institute of Japan resigned, as did the director of Tokyo Women's Medical University Hospital. The physician who supervised the surgical team and allegedly ordered a nurse and technician to cover up the error by altering diagnostic records was indicted for destroying evidence of malpractice and dismissed from the university. Other individuals who were not involved, including the director of the university, surrendered a portion of their salaries. At a press conference, the director said, "These workers caused the public to lose faith in medical treatment by committing acts—such as destroying evidence—that should never be committed by those entrusted with other people's lives."

Underlying these public actions to make amends for a grievous failure is an implied covenant between health care providers and the people who come to them for healing. If medical errors are to be prevented, the health care system will have to establish a new covenant whereby patients who are harmed are not shut out or discarded but elevated to a special status.

How can health care organizations make the transformation from denial and secrecy to honesty and openness? Leadership from the CEO and senior management of a health care organization can change the whole atmosphere. A former CEO of a large health system describes how he became aware of the need for his health system to work to make medical mistakes as rare as they can be. He admits, "I was pretty much like others and lulled into complacency. But then I attended a program with leaders on the medical error issue and realized that for too long, I relied on individual incident reports that came across my desk and never realized that if you aggregate all the errors that occur around the country, it's a huge problem. What other part of our society would allow a 747 to go down every day?"

The CEO began working with his board and senior management and spent a year educating them. The board had to realize that more incident reports would appear, which is not a bad thing, and means that the honesty policy is working. The mistakes that were kept hidden behind the wall would be surfacing.

Meanwhile, the unions were uneasy and concerned that their members would suffer punitive action if they reported a mistake or near miss. Fear of punitive action is a very real fear for many nurses, pharmacists, technicians, and others, especially for those whose work environments are unsupportive. This CEO made a point of getting involved in every incident and spoke personally with the staff involved. He didn't ask, "Who did it?" He asked, "What did we do wrong?" "Where did the process fall down?" "Is the support system in place for the family and the caregiver?" Word spread fast throughout the health system that it was a new day.

The CEO tells how the new honesty policy played out in the case of a young boy who was involved in an accident and brought to the emergency room of a local hospital in his system. The boy was in serious condition, and his brain was swelling. A medication was prescribed, but a mistake was made when a verbal order for the medication was given over the phone, and a few extra zeroes were added to the dose. The patient died, and at first, it wasn't clear whether the cause was the initial injury or the drug overdose. The CEO said the family should be told about the overdose irrespective of whether it caused the little boy's death. The family was informed and told how and where things broke down. The nurse who added the zeros felt terrible; because the hospital is located in a small community, the nurse personally knew the family. Deeply moved by how devastated she was, the family reached out to comfort her. The CEO reflects on this tragedy and says, "This medication error wasn't her fault. With all the technology we have today, why are we giving verbal orders over the phone?"

■ ■ ■

Mahatma Gandhi's words are apropos of patients, especially those who have suffered harm. A patient can best be viewed as "the most important visitor on our premises. He may be dependent on us, but we are also dependent on him. He is not an interruption to our work. He is the purpose of it. He is not an outsider to our work, he is central to it. We are not doing him a favor by serving him. He is doing us a favor by giving us the opportunity to serve him."

Health care organizations have a special opportunity and moral obligation to serve patients who have been harmed. Elevating them and their families to a special status is the only way out of an otherwise adversarial, inhumane, costly, and brutal process that, ironically, all started from the very human desire to be healed.

12 | Taking Matters into Their Own Hands

Many who are harmed by medical mistakes are abandoned by the doctors who treated them, and they are left to fend for themselves to find another doctor who can repair the damage. Victims and their families may spend years trying to hold people accountable for the harm caused, realizing that if they themselves can be harmed, so can someone else. Medical bills can mount into the thousands, if not hundreds of thousands, of dollars. As Daniel, the former White House official who became disabled after catastrophic damage to his face, says, "I feel like I have to pay my torturers." Some patients and families exhaust all their resources in trying to overcome their tragedy and must declare bankruptcy.

Here you'll read more about some of the people you have met, and we'll introduce you to new people who have taken matters into their own hands. Some intervened to save their loved one's life or their own. Others took charge by delving into their medical records to try to learn what went wrong. You'll meet people who, in the aftermath of a medical mistake, decided whether or not to seek legal redress in the courts. Sometimes the decision is not theirs to make because legislatures have enacted barriers to people using the courts to air their grievances and seek redress—barriers that add salt to still-fresh wounds.

Repairing the Damage

FAMILIES TAKE CHARGE

John and his family took matters into their own hands when they witnessed the poor care their mother, Beth, was receiving for a serious heart ailment. The hospital discharged Beth to a nursing home without discussing discharge options with the family. John, a university teacher, says he believed that the nursing home intended to keep his mother on a respirator because it would receive higher reimbursement. "I was very troubled because I knew that if my mother remained in the nursing home on a respirator, without any effort to wean her from it and restore her health, she would have died a slow, horrible death," he recalls. "She once led a vibrant life, making holiday meals for our large family and visiting her grandchildren and was suddenly treated as if she were incompetent and senile when, in fact, she wasn't."

The family contacted an air ambulance service and paid $10,000 to fly their mother, along with a respiratory therapist and registered nurse, from the nursing home in New York to an out-of-state rehabilitation hospital. There, she received the necessary rehabilitation therapy and was weaned off the respirator. About a year later, Beth went back to live independently in her own home in New York. She has regained her life and is able to drive, go to all her community and church activities, and see her grandchildren's graduations.

Even when patients and families take charge and do all that is humanly possible to help their loved one, it still may not be enough to shield them from preventable mistakes that harm them. Doctors are not immune either, and they bear the consequences of mistakes even with their knowledge and membership in the same tribe. In fact, 35 percent of physicians surveyed reported errors in the care they or their family members had received; 7 percent of those surveyed reported that the errors resulted in serious injury, including death.[1]

A pediatrician from Kansas City, who was nationally recognized for his work in medical ethics, described a devastating experience when he was hospitalized for cancer. He told his story on Bill Moyers' PBS documentary, *"On Our Own Terms."* He recalled being wheeled down to the X-ray room, where "I was left in a hallway all by myself, crying and trying to get people . . . to call the nurse and get me back to my room. I had been without pain medication for several hours. Nobody seemed to take that very seriously. And if you didn't take pain in a full professor in your medical school very seriously, you can imagine how not seriously you take it for everybody else." The physician later died from cancer.

Physicians who end up on the other side of the bedrails often are stripped of their status when they enter the hospital. They wear the same loose cloth gowns with open-air seating as everyone else. They join the ranks of other patients. If doctors can be held hostage to a system that is out of their control, and they can be treated this way, imagine what happens to a person with no family, no advocate, and no insurance. The lesson here is that even doctors often are unable to take matters into their own knowledgeable and skilled hands to prevent substandard care and medical mistakes from happening to them.

SALVAGE SURGEONS

When patients suffer from surgical and other mistakes and survive, they may need to come to their own rescue, if they are able, and find someone who has the skill to perform the corrective surgery they need. One young woman, Kim, described having to find a surgeon to correct the damage done after surgery for ulcerative colitis, an inflammatory bowel disorder that causes sores, or ulcers, in the lining of the large intestine. While trying to create a new large intestine, the surgeon punctured Kim's reproductive tract. She said, "After the surgery, I had a bowel movement and it came out of the wrong opening in my body. The nurse just stood there and said,

'Oh, my God.'" The surgeon was called and he performed emergency surgery.

After the emergency surgery, Kim was determined to find a doctor who was competent. She went to her gynecologist to see if he knew an expert who could fix what had happened. Referring to the original surgeon, her gynecologist told her, "Don't let him touch you."

Kim eventually got an appointment with a doctor at a nationally known facility. When she met with him, Kim realized she had finally found a competent surgeon who was the "sweetest guy." He referred to himself as a "salvage surgeon," which means he repairs the work of general surgeons who are performing procedures they don't know how to do. Kim says, "There are so many doctors who have the God complex, but they don't know what they are doing." Now living with a temporary ileostomy, which is a surgically created opening in the wall of the abdomen through which digested food passes, Kim says she is now reasonably comfortable with it. It lasts about ten years and will eventually have to be replaced with a permanent one. But she is not looking forward to going under anesthesia again. "I worry—am I going to wake up the next time?"

When patients such as Kim have conditions such as bowel disorders, it can be embarrassing to talk about them because they are so personal. But she advises, "Don't be ashamed. It's your body. I know there are people who are meek and who curl up in a ball and let people kick them when they are down." Kim is surely not one of those, and her courage has lessons for us all. "Don't think your life is so horrendous that you can't make it through the next day. Take one day at a time."

Some people are lucky enough to have personal friends who are surgeons. Such a friend came to the rescue of Dick, a seventy-seven-year-old retired store manager and now, along with his wife, a hospice volunteer. As part of his efforts to stay healthy, Dick was conscientious about obtaining proper preventive care, so at his doctor's suggestion, he went for a routine colonoscopy. After the procedure, the doctor came out of the room and described to Dick's wife, Jeanne, what he had done and then added nonchalantly, "Oh, by the way, your husband is in a lot of pain, and I've called an ambulance."

At the hospital, several tests were conducted, and they came back negative for perforation of the bowel, a known complication of a colonoscopy. The pain was caused by gas, Jeanne was repeatedly told. But the pain was increasing, and the fever worsening. Another X-ray was taken about twelve hours after the colonoscopy and showed that the bowel had indeed been perforated. Surgery was performed right away and revealed massive peritonitis.

The doctor told Jeanne that it was time to call all the children to their father's bedside, as Dick was inches from death. The large Irish-Catholic family assembled from all corners of the country. But because Dick had been in good physical condition for a man of his age, and, as his wife says, because of the family's prayers, he pulled through and lived.

Dick was willing to tolerate the colostomy that was the result of the initial surgery because, as he says, "No way, I don't want to go through any surgery again"—a common reaction of many patients who are so afraid after already having suffered medical mishaps. "It was on my mind that something would go wrong again. One night while I was in the hospital, one of the many bad dreams I had was of a doctor who was doing an autopsy on me. I was trying to shout, 'Don't cut me, I'm still here!'"

After Dick was out of danger and at home for a while, a family friend who is a surgeon called him at home on a Saturday morning. He told Dick, "Come in Monday morning, I'll take care of the colostomy for you." Dick trusted this longtime friend who came to the rescue, and had the colostomy reversed. It has now been three years since Dick's brush with death, and he is doing pretty well. He says with a grin that he has gained most of the weight back that he had lost.

Setting the Record Straight

Some patients and families take matters into their own hands by poring over their medical records, and what they read can be surprising if not shocking. In the aftermath of her son's death, Ilene recalls that one of the doctors who examined her son denied ever doing so. Sure enough, there was no record of the visit Michael had made to the doctor. But the doctor had written a prescription for him that day, and the pharmacy had that prescription with his signature on it. After Michael died, Ilene went to the pharmacy to obtain a copy of it.

When Diana, the former Air Force Intelligence Officer, obtained a copy of her voluminous medical records documenting her long and tortuous experience in the health care system, she was amazed at what she found. The orthopedic surgeon who operated on her hip wrote in her medical record a lengthy commentary describing her as a "histrionic patient chronically dissatisfied and demanding attention" and "unable to accept competent medical care." It is no coincidence, she believes, that this note was written after she wrote to the president of the hospital that was so ill equipped and understaffed to meet even her most basic needs, requesting a transfer to another hospital. The doctor who wrote the note had recently been promoted to chief of staff of that hospital, and no doubt her letter did not shine a favorable light on the performance of this physician in his new role. Reflecting on the doctor's power to "edit vital documentation to portray a patient in an unfavorable light, influencing others who read it," she says, "he can skew and misrepresent treatment notes with an eye to discrediting the patient." By discrediting the patient in the medical record, the doctor protects himself in the event of a malpractice suit and makes it extraordinarily difficult for patients to have any hope of holding doctors accountable for negligent care.

A husband whose wife was dying from cancer that had been undiagnosed was furious that the cancer had been missed. In the waning days of his wife's life, he and his daughter went to his wife's

primary care doctor; tempers were raging at the thought that someone they dearly loved was dying because the cancer was not diagnosed until it was much too late. A former critical care nurse, his
wife had dutifully gone for her regular checkups, yet the cancer had
been missed. Her husband insisted on seeing the doctor and
demanded his wife's medical records. Realizing that the husband
was a force to be reckoned with, the doctor handed over the medical records. The family made a copy and returned the original.

His daughter reviewed them with a fine eye and found consultant reports dated several years earlier that suggested the possibility of cancer and recommended further evaluation. The wife's
primary care physician of almost twenty years never followed up.
The cancer was diagnosed only when she went to the hospital in a
great deal of pain, but by then it was far too late. The cancer had
spread and was rampant throughout her body. She died about a
month after the cancer was finally diagnosed.

Working Together

The mother whose eighteen-month-old girl, Josie, died as a result of
miscommunication and systems failure in a prestigious East Coast
hospital, didn't take her daughter's death sitting down. Soon after the
tragedy, and in the midst of her anger and grief, Josie's mother, Sorrel, challenged the hospital to do the right thing by establishing a
paient safety program named after Josie, the Josie King Patient Safety
Institute. One of its goals is to change the culture of the hospital so
there is greater openness in talking about errors and near misses and
meaningful actions taken to prevent them.

Sorrel is working with a physician at the hospital who is nationally recognized for his work to prevent errors. Together, they are
teaching medical students and hospital staff about the perils of
miscommunication with family members and among members of
the different health care tribes. Sorrel and the doctor did grand
rounds at the hospital, and it was standing room only, a sign that

Josie's death was a wake-up call. As part of the patient safety program named for Josie, a culture of safety is being established on two floors of the children's hospital.

Meanwhile, Sorrel is invited to speak to audiences of doctors, nurses, hospital administrators, and others around the country about the tragedy that has altered her life forever and about the urgent need for change. She tells them, "This problem is unlike cancer, AIDS, or other diseases where we must wait for a scientific breakthrough. Hospital errors are a man-made epidemic. Doctors and nurses make mistakes, and lives are being lost. You are the only ones that can solve this problem—not lawyers, not insurance companies, and not people like me."

To Sue or Not to Sue

People who sue doctors and hospitals are often perceived as just trying to win a lottery by filing "frivolous" lawsuits. The fact is that most people who are harmed do not sue. Moreover, taking a closer look and listening to why some people do take legal action, it's clear that there is no frivolity motivating them to seek legitimate redress for harm that has been done.

When we asked Kim why she sued the doctor and hospital where the original surgery was performed, she describes how her life changed after the original surgery. "Because I had twelve consecutive months on medical leave, I was fired from my job as a quality assurance technician. My husband had to take a lot of time off from work because of my illness, and he lost his job. He was in international shipping and receiving, and the events of September eleventh slowed things down, but while some people were eventually called back, he wasn't.

"We lost our house and had to foreclose. We lived with my brother and his wife in their house on a farm for a while, but field mice came into the house, and I couldn't live there. We ended up staying with my mom—my husband, myself, and two kids—and we slept on the living room floor."

Kim says she can't get back what she has already lost. "I'm not looking to win the lottery. It's just to rebuild. And I want the doctor to acknowledge what he did. I want him to say that he is sorry and that he means it."

Another woman shared a similar experience. She is in the middle of litigation and cannot share many details of her story, another manifestation of the wall of silence. She was in her twenties when she underwent an elective procedure that was supposed to last only forty minutes, but her life was forever changed. She says, "I used to have a really good job but can't work any more because I have to stay near the bathroom most days—sometimes I have to go thirty times a day. I don't have a way to earn an income. The pain is like having labor pains in your colon. I went through a year of vomiting excrement and lost a lot of my teeth because of it. There's more than $10,000 in dental bills that have to be paid.

"We are not suing to get a new swimming pool. I lost my entire large intestine, and my small intestine doesn't work the way it should. The doctor who did this to me had done this procedure before, I later found out, and made similar mistakes. He shouldn't be doing these any more."

She continues, "The worst days are when I am really sick and my daughter notices, and she brushes my hair and rubs my face. The absolute worst is when I am sleeping next to the toilet, and she comes in and lays down beside me."

Medical mistakes can bring financial ruin, and it's reasonable for people harmed to want to be compensated. A husband whose wife died because of a hospital-acquired infection resulting from very poor infection control had medical bills that eventually approached $1 million for the more than four hundred days his wife was in the hospital being treated for the infection; the bills stopped coming only after he initiated legal proceedings. For

Susan, who incurred medical bills after her doctor failed to take action when she developed a life-threatening infection after laparoscopic surgery, legal action was the only recourse available to her to pay the bills she charged to her credit card. She also wanted to recoup the expenses her mother incurred when she made several trips from the Midwest to care for her.

Living with the disabling and painful effects of medical mistakes, some survivors don't have the energy to pursue legal action. Mary, the television anchor whom you met earlier, did not pursue legal action, even though the medical mistake caused her to lose her house and her livelihood, and her bills mount into the thousands every month. "I had only so much energy, and I had to use it just to survive," she says.

Other victims and family members can't bear the thought of years of legal wrangling that can have an uncertain outcome. If they lose the case, they may, in turn, be sued by the doctor for costs incurred in a defense. One family whose loved one died from an alleged medical mistake was too "petrified" to talk publicly or privately; the doctor, who they said missed a life-threatening diagnosis, sued the family, who was of modest means, and a lien was placed on their house and the future financial assets of their children.

Do doctors think patients should sue if medical mistakes result in harm? More than half of physicians who were surveyed think so. The survey, conducted by researchers at the Harvard School of Public Health, asked physicians and the public whether a doctor should be sued for malpractice when a patient dies after being prescribed and administered a medication to which the patient has a known allergy that is noted in the medical record. The survey findings were published in the *New England Journal of Medicine* and revealed that 55 percent of physicians believe that a doctor should be sued in a case such as this, while a higher percentage of the public—69 percent—said they thought the doctor should be sued.[2]

FROM PATIENT TO PLAINTIFF

When patients are harmed, and there is no honesty or account-ability, the legal recourse they and their families seek is not for the faint of heart. "There's a harshness and brutality in a trial, says Justin's mother. "They ask you about your marriage—as if that has anything to do with the fact that my son died because his condi-tion was misdiagnosed in the emergency room. I was forty-eight years old when this happened, and there I was one day in this huge room with all these attorneys. I asked myself, 'What am I doing here? My child died, and I am having to go through this?' They just try to wear you down. My lawyer said he was afraid the trial would kill me. And I told him that I'm afraid the trial *won't* kill me and I'll have to keep on living."

Elizabeth's mom, Leila, described how she wanted to ensure that her daughter would have some financial security now that she is permanently paralyzed. "It is a sick system. To the attorneys, it is a deal. To me, it's my daughter's life and her future when she will be disabled all of her life." Leila is very well aware that the system doesn't mind dragging on cases for a prolonged period. If the child dies, the cost to the doctors and hospitals at settlement time is less in dollars and cents than if the child lives with a significant dis-ability.

For those who do try to pursue legal action, the results can be inexplicable to family members. A judge dismissed a case brought forward by a daughter whose mother died from sub-standard care and errors. Seven years later, the daughter still has so many questions, "Why did the attorney, who promised me there would be justice and that my mother didn't die in vain, abandon me and withdraw from the case? Why were the defense attorneys paid so much money to defend the providers who made the mistake? Why wasn't anyone interested in the truth, which could have been used to save someone else's life in the future?"

SILENCED AGAIN

Pursuing litigation can have the perverse effect of accomplishing the opposite of what most patients and families want: a voice. When people who have been harmed by mistakes pursue legal recourse, their lawyers often tell them that they shouldn't discuss the case publicly or even privately with other victims who can give advice and support on the treacherous and lonely road to justice. Patients and families may feel compelled to agree to gag orders in settlement agreements, which is another way that the truth about medical errors remains behind the wall of silence.

The husband whose wife died from an infection in a Connecticut hospital, and who used the courts to force the hospital to disclose its poor infection control practices, faced another encounter with the hospital. He talked to a newspaper reporter who was writing a story about the spiraling number of hospital deaths from hospital-acquired infections, and the published story mentioned the tragedy that befell this widower in his seventies. A few days later, the hospital where his wife died sued him, claiming that he violated the terms of his settlement agreement. The husband said clearly, "I never broke the terms of the settlement. I never said how much they paid me, which is the only thing I couldn't say."

A flurry of negative publicity against the hospital ensued because of its harsh treatment against a man who had lost his wife due to the hospital's own negligence. A local newspaper compared the hardball tactics of the hospital with those used by the Catholic Church to silence victims of sexual abuse. Faced with the backlash, the hospital retreated and withdrew the lawsuit. Courageously standing his ground, the widower says, "You have to fight these people. They threaten you, but if you know you are right, you can't give up." When asked where his courage came from to battle it out with the hospital, he says with gusto, "It's probably from being a Sicilian, my parents were born there."

Challenging the system may be out of the question for people who are completely dependent on it—even if they have experienced the effects of a medical error. This is what happened to a veteran who was cared for at the Lexington VA medical center. In an account by Dr. Kraman, the chief of staff of the medical center, a seventy-two-year-old veteran became blind in one eye in part because of poor advice that his wife was given when she reported that her husband was having periodic episodes of blindness.[3] The veteran's primary care physician informed the medical center's risk management committee about the man's blindness, and after a thorough review of the care provided, the committee concluded that he did not receive appropriate care. Because of the medical center's humane and ethical disclosure policy, the husband and wife were informed about the poor care. They received an apology, and amends were made. Only then did they admit that they believed the blindness was the result of the poor care the husband was given. They were afraid to speak up because they feared the husband would lose his veteran's benefits.

IT'S NOT ABOUT THE MONEY

For many families who are successful in pursuing whatever justice the legal system can muster, the motivation is not about the money. It can never make up for the loss of a loved one's life, a limb, or the ability to walk again. When family members receive a check in the mail or in a lawyer's office, it can be an emotional and confusing time; money is hardly compensation for a loss of someone or something for which there can never be any compensation. It is society's feeble attempt to make amends in the face of tragedy, and is a poor proxy for accountability. Some families say it is immoral to put a dollar amount on a life, but that is what the legal system does. To find meaning in what is otherwise a crude exchange, some of the people whom you have met have used the proceeds from settlements for a higher purpose that does honor to the memory of their loved one.

One family whose son died from a medical mistake used the proceeds from a settlement with the hospital to support initiatives to prevent medical mistakes. A woman in California whose mother died from a medical mistake used the money to go to law school to acquire the skills to be an effective advocate for patients and families—which she has become. A grandmother is using the proceeds she received after the death of her husband to send her grandchild to medical school. The Connecticut husband whose wife died from the hospital-acquired infection used part of the proceeds from the settlement with the hospital to bring his brother-in-law's body back from Europe, where he died in World War II, so he could be buried next to his sister.

One mother wonders why people have to go to court to receive compensation in cases where everyone admits a terrible mistake occurred. She says, "I found it astonishing that no one from the hospital ever contacted us with any offer of settlement despite the fact that the doctors had admitted fault. It is a scandal that people are forced to resort to litigation to receive compensation for egregious medical errors. You cannot imagine the revulsion that a family feels at the idea of negotiating a price for the life of a loved one. It is barbaric. In many cases, as in ours, what people really want is an acknowledgment, a correction, and a legacy."

MORE WALLS OF SILENCE

Some who have suffered from medical mistakes cannot take legal action because state legislatures, in passing tort reform legislation, impose barriers that are impossible to overcome. You read earlier about the husband whose wife died from cancer that was not diagnosed for several years. The state where he lives has a three-year statute of limitations on medical malpractice suits, and the clock starts ticking when the mistake happens. In this case, the clock started ticking when the possibility of cancer was noted in a consultant's report. The report had been placed in the wife's medical record a couple of years before the rampant cancer was diagnosed. Her primary care physician never followed up on the consultant's recommendation for further evaluation. The husband says, "By the time you realize they made a mistake in diagnosing the cancer when it was possibly treatable, it's too late to take any action and hold anyone accountable. How can a law that puts a statute of limitations in place like that be considered reform?"

Many of the people and families you have read about in this book are deeply anguished by a vote in the U.S. House of Representatives in March 2003 in support of legislation to limit the ability of patients and families to obtain redress when errors occur. The bill would cap medical malpractice awards for pain and suffering at $250,000. Malpractice cases can be costly to undertake, and in many instances, the costs to lawyers outweigh the returns they receive. As a consequence, patients and families often find it difficult to obtain legal representation—and to have the opportunity to hold the health care system accountable for errors that result in serious injury and death. As of this writing, the bill is being considered in the U.S. Senate. Any medical malpractice reform needs to account for people who have been harmed. Will society turn a blind eye to the suffering of those who have already suffered beyond what most people can imagine?

In the prime of his life and with many years of robust earnings ahead were it not for his medically induced disability, Daniel, the former White House official, has after nine years been unable to receive any compensation for the injuries he sustained, the income he lost because he has not been able to work, the future income he will lose because of his disability, and the hundreds of thousands of dollars of medical expenses he has had to pay. If it weren't for family resources, he says, his medically induced disability would have been a "death sentence after a period of torture." Living in "near-constant agony," Daniel says, "I wish our lawmakers could enact legislation to limit my suffering and the suffering of others. Since they cannot do this, they should not limit our ability to recover what can never adequately be recovered. It only hurts people who are trying to live against all odds."

If Daniel, who is in his prime earning years, has been unable to obtain compensation for the harm he has suffered, imagine the experience of others who are egregiously harmed who are not in the prime income-generating years—retirees, stay-at-home mothers, and children. They are even more likely to be shut out of any opportunity to obtain compensation because they generate no income and their lives have less economic value in the eyes of the courts. What happens to them if they don't have the resources to pay for a roof over their heads or medical care to repair the damage?

Here's another consideration missed in the medical malpractice debate. If medical malpractice is viewed as simply a dispute between two parties—the patient who was allegedly harmed and the health care provider accused of causing harm—there may be more to it than that. If the care a doctor or hospital provides to a patient is negligent and does not meet the standard of care, and if such care is allowed to continue to be rendered with impunity, future patients in that community may be at risk for harm.

Real Medical Malpractice Reform

Real medical malpractice reform has nothing to do with the rising cost of doctors' medical malpractice insurance premiums. Nor does it have anything to do with the political battles between the health care industry and trial lawyers. The patients' voice is lost in the din of the wrangling of special interests—when in fact, the real special interests should be those of patients and families, who are best represented by their own voice, and no one else's.

Real malpractice reform would make medical mistakes as rare as possible. It would establish a system of checks and balances that brings accountability for errors to the doorstep of the health care facilities where they happen. Helen, who lost her son Lewis to medical error, eloquently states the level of accountability that is needed. "Serious error needs to be rare enough that hospitals feel the need, as other industries do now, to fall all over themselves trying to make it up to the customer when something does go awry."

This is the real reform agenda and speaks from the hearts and minds of those who aren't fighting for their own self-interest. They have nothing to gain financially from the outcome of any legislative action. It's an agenda that will help not just a select few, but every American. Their motive is about as pure as it can be. Who in Washington can say that?

13 | Brick by Brick:
Tearing Down the Wall

Many of the people and families you have met have ideas that would make errors as rare as possible. This chapter gives voice to some of their ideas, as well as others. They are the most motivated to prevent errors because they know firsthand their impact. It's one thing to lose a loved one, or a part of one's body, or the capability to do everyday things because of disease or injury; it is an entirely different matter to sustain such a loss because of a preventable mistake. Reforms need to be made as if people's lives depended on it, because they do.

Do Ask, *Do* Tell

In a $1.5 trillion health care system, hospitals, like any other business, need to be accountable for providing services that don't harm the people they serve. The frequency of serious medical mistakes is an indicator of how well—or how poorly— hospitals are working to keep patients free from harm. It is reasonable for the public to expect that health care organizations are doing everything they can to prevent errors. If this expectation isn't fulfilled, it is also reasonable for the public to expect that the government, which pays a large percentage of America's health care bill, should exercise its oversight functions to ensure that the public's health is in good hands.

For the foreseeable future, the American public won't know if the health care industry is doing this part of its job because it is resisting the mandatory reporting of serious errors that result in death and injury. The industry is concerned that such reporting will lead to more lawsuits, while individual hospitals are concerned that public reporting of medical mistakes will hurt their reputations.

The protectionist arguments no longer carry any weight. When the lives of thousands of people are at stake, the collective good trumps the right of private organizations to withhold information that affects the public's health. Imagine if the airline industry didn't want to report serious injuries and deaths from airplane crashes.

Keeping Score

Here's why reporting of errors—or keeping score—is so important. Imagine if a spate of plane crashes occurred in which several hundred passengers died, and Congress asked airline industry executives to testify in a Congressional hearing on what the industry was doing to make air travel safer. Imagine further that the only information airline industry executives could report about the number of deaths from crashes was about ten to twenty years old! Outdated information about the safety of air travel simply would not be tolerated. But this is the exact situation that exists when it comes to the safety of health care. The IOM's estimates of deaths from medical errors were based primarily on a study that reviewed the medical records of patients who were hospitalized in New York in 1984 and on the Utah and Colorado study that examined the care of patients hospitalized in those states in 1992. This is the best information that exists at the present time. No new studies are under way to document the number of medical errors nationwide or to track whether the number of errors is increasing, decreasing, or staying the same.

Let's take another example closer to home. Imagine if no one kept score at all the football, baseball, and soccer games held around the country every year. Baseball fans wouldn't know whether a team is playing better or worse with the new pitcher that was just hired for millions of dollars. Coaches and players would have no incentive to win if no one is keeping score.

And so it is with medical mistakes. No one is keeping score. Imagine a team that didn't want to be scored, and all the major league teams agreed. What would sports fans say about them? It probably wouldn't be fit to print, but at a minimum, fans would probably say the teams aren't serious about winning—or even trying to win. They just want to take the ticket proceeds and go home.

As in sports, if there's no score-keeping on the safety of health care, the public will never know whether it is going with a winning health care team or a losing one. Sports fans can walk away from games, but people who are sick cannot walk away from what may be the only hospital in town. Just because health care isn't an option for people who are sick, that doesn't mean they should be captive to those who don't want to keep score.

As the IOM recommended, hospitals should be required to collect information on when the system breaks down—that is, when medical mistakes occur that result in death or serious injury—and report this information to public agencies. The place to start is the list of "never events" developed by the National Quality Forum with input from many health care experts.

The first step should be for hospitals to report even a few of the twenty-seven different events, including surgery conducted on the wrong patient or the wrong part of the body, objects left in patients during surgery, and blood transfusions using the wrong blood type.

Will this information help the public know which hospitals are safer than others? Hospitals that report consistently high error rates as compared with their peers might be doing a less than stellar job of proactively avoiding medical mistakes, and the public would come to know this. On the other hand, old habits die hard, and some hospitals might be reluctant to report errors, which will make the conscientious facilities that do accurately report errors look as if they have more errors when, in fact, they are just being honest.

The advantage of using the "never events" as a starting point is that the mistakes are obvious, and patients and families are likely to know when they occur and can independently report them, which can serve as a built-in check on whether hospitals are accurately reporting errors. If conscientious doctors and nurses could confidentially report such errors as well—not just for internal quality improvement but also for accountability—another checkpoint would be in place.

It's important to bear in mind that the "never events" are just some of the indicators that can be used to determine whether a hospital is doing a good job of taking care of patients—safely. Other indicators, such as infection rates and whether patients with heart attacks get certain medications known to reduce mortality, are examples of other indicators of quality.

Will the public use this information? Many people probably won't. But that's not the point. Most airline travelers don't check the FAA's Web site for the safety records of airlines before booking flights. Most people don't want to know all the details of one airline versus another or which airplanes are more susceptible to rudder malfunctions than others. But they do want to know that *somebody* knows, *is* watching, and *is* enforcing the rules. This is how it works in aviation, but not in health care.

The Weakest Link

Right now, the weakest link is knowing to whom hospitals will report errors, what will happen to the information they report, and whether there will be sufficient oversight and enforcement so hospitals take corrective action when needed.

You'll recall from earlier that only twenty states have mandatory reporting of errors, and very few errors are reported. States' health departments don't have adequate funding or staff to collect, analyze, investigate, and report medical mistakes. It will take years to build that capacity—assuming the states have the political will and the money to fund it. Appropriations from state legislatures will be subject to the whims of states' budgets and open to influence from health industry lobbying. Even if funding were available, it would never be equitable across the states because some states are wealthier than others, and people living in states with less fiscal capacity would be deprived of oversight that protects their health.

Lessons from other industries can be instructive on how to pay for a mandatory medical error reporting system. In the aftermath of September 11, 2001, airport fees were increased by $2.50 per ticket to pay for enhanced security at airports, and these fees are reflected in the cost of airline tickets. In the telecommunications industry, long-distance telephone users pay a universal connectivity charge to fund a federal program that provides affordable telecommunications services for low-income customers and subsidizes Internet access for eligible schools and libraries.

Similarly, to pay for mandatory reporting systems, one funding option is to add a modest annual fee to the cost of health insurance premiums for every individual or family that is covered, with the proceeds earmarked for collecting, analyzing, and publicly reporting medical errors. Another option is to add a modest fee to the cost of every hospital admission—a less desirable option because it disproportionately affects those who are sick enough to be hospitalized. Once a fee-based approach is in place, it is less subject to the whim of annual appropriations in Congress or state legislatures, and to tinkering by the health care industry. The public would be supportive if they knew the proceeds from the fees would be used to make health care safer.

Bear or Bull?

Even with mandatory reporting of all twenty-seven "never events" the public still won't know in 2009, ten years after the IOM report, whether another million people will have died from medical mistakes in the first decade of the twenty-first century. While mandatory reporting of some mistakes gets under way, another study should be conducted that uses the same methodology as that used in the two studies cited in the IOM report to determine whether medical mistakes are becoming more rare or more frequent. We now have a baseline of as many as 98,000 deaths every year from medical mistakes in hospitals. The public has a right to know whether this number is increasing, decreasing, or staying the same.

Which Team Is a Winning Team?

In the previous chapter, you read about Dick, the retired store manager whose colon was perforated during a routine colonoscopy. His wife, Jeanne, says she wishes she and her husband had known more about the doctor who performed the colonoscopy. While perforation of the bowel is a known complication associated with the procedure, patients don't know how many colonoscopies a doctor performs, nor his or her complication rate. Dick says, "You need to know how many of these things happen on his watch, even if he is board-certified, so you can make a decent decision on who to go with."

If a doctor has a much higher rate of bowel perforation, it might be a sign of more than just a lot of usual complications and an indication that the doctor is not sufficiently trained or skilled to perform the procedure. In Dick's case, the colonoscopy was performed in a physician's office—where there is no government oversight to ensure that a physician is trained or certified before starting to perform such procedures on patients. A high rate of complications could signal preventable perforations and, therefore, medical mistakes. Without information that tracks the number of procedures and complication rates by physician, it's virtually impossible to determine when complications really are errors because the doctor is unskilled.

Very little information exists to answer Dick's questions—how many procedures are done, and what's the outcome for the patient? The New York State Department of Health has led the country in providing information to the public about mortality rates from coronary artery bypass surgery performed in hospitals in the state. It set the gold standard by developing a list of mortality rates for each hospital and for each doctor who performs the surgery. The mortality rates are adjusted so that doctors and hospitals that treat patients who are less healthy are not at a disadvantage when their performance is compared with that of other doctors and hospitals whose patients might be healthier.

So, for example, the Department of Health issued a report in November 2002 with risk-adjusted mortality rates for the approximately 18,000 cardiac bypass surgeries performed each year in thirty-three hospitals in the state. The mortality rates in hospitals range from a high of seven deaths per 100 patients to a low of less than one death per 100 patients. Overall, there has been nearly a 36 percent decline in mortality rates associated with cardiac bypass surgery since 1989, when the Department of Health first began reporting surgery outcomes. What is the lesson here? When hospitals and surgeons can compare their performance with that of their peers, it gives them an incentive to improve the survival rates for their patients. Some hospitals that had higher mortality rates than their peers stopped performing bypass surgery. Others kept their doors open and hired a new surgical team.

The number of deaths from surgery declined, some experts say, because doctors stopped operating on very sick patients, who are at higher risk of dying during or after surgery. Others suggest that the number of people who died from heart attacks overall increased slightly because the sicker patients had less chance of finding a surgeon who would operate because a high-risk patient could reflect poorly on the physician's track record. But the bottom line is that information was made available that showed the difference between a hospital with a good track record and one that was less good.

Yet do people facing the prospect of bypass surgery use this information when making decisions on who should perform the surgery and in which hospital? The truth is that many of them don't. The main reason is that they don't know such information exists, and little effort is made to make the information available to those who need it most, a problem that is not insurmountable. Also, many patients don't choose their heart surgeon or hospital. They are more likely to get a referral from their primary care or other doctor. So the choice may not be theirs to make.

Knowing the mortality rates for a particular procedure—by hospital and doctor—is the bottom line for many patients and families. The California legislature enacted a law in 2001 requiring its Department of Health Services to collect and report similar information on mortality rates from heart bypass surgery and other medical procedures. Consumers Union is at the table in this process to help ensure that the public has ready access to information that is easily understandable. Other states have a long way to go to provide the same information to the public.

In the interim, how well patients are cared for can be determined by information on some key indicators. In December 2002, the American Hospital Association announced that hospitals will voluntarily report how well they care for patients with conditions such as heart attacks, congestive heart failure, and pneumonia. Hospitals will track and publicize certain indicators of the quality of care that have been found to increase the likelihood that patients come out of the hospital alive. For example, experts recommend that heart attack patients should receive beta-blockers, yet too few do. The quality indicators will help the public—and other hospitals—compare performance among different facilities. The voluntary aspect of this initiative, though, still allows quality improvement to be optional—when it shouldn't.

"Sunlight Is the Best Disinfectant"

Another indicator of system breakdown in hospitals is a high rate of hospital-acquired infections. You read earlier about the woman who died in a Connecticut hospital after acquiring an infection as a result of the hospital's exceedingly poor infection control practices. Her husband took the hospital to court to force it to reveal its infection control records to the public. He won, and the hospital was required by the state's Supreme Court to open its internal files for public scrutiny. The hospital worked very hard to reduce its infection rate and now proudly reports a very low infection rate—a win-win for the hospital and all the patients who are treated there. While opening its records to the public was no doubt bitter medicine for the hospital, it was necessary medicine that reduces the risk to people living in the community who might be hospitalized at that facility. Former U.S. Supreme Court Justice Brandeis was right when he wrote almost ninety years ago, "Sunlight is said to be the best of disinfectants."

Does it make sense for individual patients and family members to take each of the 5,000 hospitals individually to court to require hospitals to report infection rates publicly? It doesn't make sense. Hospital-acquired infections affect 2 million people each year, according to the Centers for Disease Control and Prevention (CDC). About 300 hospitals are working voluntarily with the CDC on a national hospital infection surveillance system, which started in 1970. It is a confidential and voluntary hospital-based reporting system that monitors infections that patients can succumb to while they are hospitalized and guides efforts to prevent them. Not surprisingly, participating hospitals have reported lower infection rates because of effective monitoring and prevention. With 5,000 short-term general hospitals in the United States, there's a long way to go. Hospitals' infection rates should be routinely tracked and reported, and when a hospital's infection rate is an outlier and higher than its peers, this information should be publicly reported.

Truly Informed Consent

Some patients and families you have met recommend that doctors give consent forms to patients well in advance of elective procedures—at least a week—so they can be read and discussed around the kitchen table. This way, patients and families have time to ask their doctor questions they otherwise wouldn't ask or have time to think about.

Susan, whose colon was punctured during a laparoscopic procedure, says she would have wanted additional information as part of her informed consent. Looking back, she wishes she had known more about the risks, which she says were underplayed by her doctor. She wanted to better understand the complications that can occur, how they manifest themselves, and how likely they occur generally. She would have wanted to know how often the doctor had done the procedure and the frequency of complications. "I do this a lot" is not very meaningful information for a patient who is about to undergo a serious medical procedure.

No More Passing the Buck

One of the nation's leaders in medical error prevention, Dr. Lucian Leape, Adjunct Professor at the Harvard School of Public Health, told the *Boston Herald*, "Every hospital has doctors whose performance is a concern. . . . Everybody has witnessed it. But everybody insists it is someone else's problem."[1] The result is that the problem of "problem doctors" lands in the lap of patients. This should not happen.

States grant medical licenses to doctors, and in so doing, are designated to safeguard the health of the public by ensuring it is served by competent physicians who meet high ethical standards. Medical licenses are not granted by virtue of membership in a medical society. Some have suggested that medical boards be reformed in fundamental ways. While each state medical board is different, some common areas of reform can be considered. The membership of medical boards needs to be more broad-based. Influential leaders in the state who have a stake in the health of the public should be included. Business leaders who are large employers have an interest in ensuring that their employees receive health care that is rendered by competent doctors. So, too, do nonprofit organizations such as AARP, veterans' organizations, and unions that represent large segments of the population. These groups have members that include many older Americans who have more interaction with the health care system than younger patients and are at greater risk for medical mistakes.

Governors often appoint medical board members, and the selection process needs to be more transparent and not subject to the nod of the state medical society. Representatives of organizations such as those noted above can be selected by the organizations themselves. While these representatives won't have medical expertise, they will bring a perspective of the society's norms, which can guide the boards' determinations of who is fit to be granted the privilege of a license to practice medicine and the circumstances under which that privilege should be taken away.

The composition of medical boards is not the only target for reform. The process by which complaints are reviewed needs to be more transparent. The number of complaints made against individual physicians should be easily accessible to the public, along with the disposition of those complaints.

Families who have filed complaints with state medical boards are advocating that disciplinary hearings be more open to the public. In Massachusetts, a thirteen-month-old girl died from fatal brain damage while she waited overnight for surgery to drain excess fluid in her skull. The girl's father has spearheaded an effort to have a bill introduced in the Massachusetts state legislature that would require medical board hearings to be open to the public. The father—a Gulf War veteran, by the way—was excluded from the board hearing when his complaint was discussed. Hoping for serious disciplinary action, he was disappointed with the board's actions, which were only to issue letters and warnings to the doctors involved. Now a state trooper, he says, "If I had neglected my daughter the way the doctors did, I would be charged with child abuse and my child would be taken away from me." Information about the actions taken against the doctors in this case is not available on the state medical board's Web site.

Another proposed reform would allow people and their families who file a complaint with a board to be given the opportunity to make a victim impact statement during the hearings when their case is discussed. This reform would allow them to present the facts as they know them and describe the impact the event has had on their health and their lives.

To some of the people you have met in this book who have sought redress from state medical boards, it is deeply perplexing that physicians convicted of fraud and sexual misconduct are allowed to continue to hold the privilege of a medical license. It is also surprising that instances of apparent negligence seem to be of so little concern to medical boards.

With so much perplexity among members of the public who file complaints with state medical boards, it would be helpful to have open, public dialogue on the standards and criteria boards use to assess whether a physician should retain a license. The present criteria lack transparency to ordinary citizens. Simply put, patients and families don't understand the standards that guide the work of medical boards, but not for lack of trying. A public dialogue could shape current standards and narrow the chasm between the criteria that medical boards use and public expectations about the competence and ethics of physicians licensed to practice. This dialogue should happen not just within individual states, but across the country.

State medical boards need more funding to meet the public's expectations. Legitimate concerns of people who have been harmed by doctors must be responded to in a timely way. A former pilot observes how the two America West airline pilots who went through airport security smelling of alcohol had their licenses revoked by the FAA within days. In contrast, medical boards can take months, if not years, to suspend or revoke a physician's license.

Finally, all states need to have easily accessible physician profiles, as Massachusetts has done. There's no justification for some Americans to have access to this information in their state while others do not.

Who Is That in the White Coat?

In teaching hospitals where doctors in training provide a lot of the care, patients and family members often don't know who is who and the level of training they have. Is the person in the white coat a first-year resident fresh out of medical school? A senior resident? A veteran doctor? It's not easy to tell. You've read about two people in this book—Leonard, whose wife died when a resident gave her an epidural incorrectly, and Lewis, who died because of inadequate postsurgical monitoring. Leonard wants to ensure that other patients and families know when they are dealing with a doctor who is still in training.

Meanwhile, Lewis's mother, Helen, has worked to have a bill introduced in her state's legislature that would require medical students, residents, and veteran doctors to wear identification badges that clearly identify their status, including the year of medical school or postgraduate study in which they are enrolled. The bill calls for identification that is written without abbreviations and in words that are understandable to the general public. Patients must be given the name of the attending physician in charge of their care and contact information, just as people outside the hospital contact their personal physician when they need a doctor's advice.

The bill would also require that patients who are admitted into a teaching hospital, where residents may care for them, must be informed that the hospital is a training facility and told of the role the trainees have in caring for the patient. The bill would make these activities a condition of hospital licensure. But these measures don't require legislation—hospitals can incorporate these practices now without legislation.

A Constituency for Change

One of the reasons that medical mistakes have been allowed to fester is that there is no powerful constituency to advocate on behalf of people and their families who have borne the consequences of medical mistakes. The good news is that more patients and their families are speaking out about medical mistakes and are forming grassroots organizations fueled by their own dedication and late-night hours on the Internet networking with people around the country, writing letters to the editors of newspapers, and talking to their legislators. Their mission is to prevent other people from suffering the same things they have experienced. Meanwhile, mothers whose children have died because of medical mistakes have discussed establishing a group similar to Mothers Against Drunk Driving (MADD), although this one might rightly be called Mothers Against Medical Errors (MAME).

Consumer-led organizations can educate the public about how to prevent mistakes from happening to them; track errors reported by consumers and health care professionals; provide advice to families on how to cope in the aftermath of a medical mistake; inform the public about how to file a complaint with a state medical board; be the voice of people harmed by the health system; and advocate for state and federal reforms to make health care safe. By engaging national organizations—veterans' organizations, AARP, unions, nursing organizations, medical students and residents—in the cause, they can collectively work on behalf of millions of Americans to make health care safe for all.

Changing Social Norms

Will any of these efforts save lives? Telling the stories of medical errors from the perspective of those who have experienced them helps raise individual and collective awareness. Just by starting to talk about errors and the impact they have on people and their families, we can begin to change the social norms surrounding medical mistakes. What is meant by social norms?

Remember how smoking used to be commonplace everywhere—on planes and trains, in offices and restaurants? The social norm for what is acceptable about where and when it's okay to smoke has changed dramatically. Today, if a smoker lights up in a no-smoking area, a throng of nonsmokers descends upon the smoker informing him or her (kindly or not so kindly) that smoking isn't allowed. This wasn't always the case. The norms about smoking—or society's expectations of what is acceptable—have changed dramatically, and all of us are healthier because of it.

Smoking and errors are very different things. But what they have in common is that people die from them. And these deaths are preventable.

Social norms need to change within health care organizations. Errors should no longer be buried but disclosed, learned from, and prevented. The norms that are taught to the next generation of doctors and nurses, as well as future health care administrators who are now in training, need to change. Those who teach them are key to changing the future generation, so society doesn't have to wait for another whole generation to unlearn the bad habits they pick up in their formative years.

Similarly, social norms about medical errors—and what society is willing to tolerate—have to change. Many Americans feel powerless to do anything. But the ace in the hole is that people are dying preventable deaths and sustaining painful injuries in great numbers. The American public is just beginning to realize that medical errors occur in large numbers, and the next step is for society to declare that these large numbers of preventable deaths and injuries are simply unacceptable.

An Aviation Analogy

Imagine if the Federal Aviation Administration didn't exist, and no one was in charge of airline safety, and as many as 100,000 people were dying each year in plane crashes. What would we as a society do?

Imagine that we started by relying on Fortune 500 companies, whose employees fly frequently, to use their purchasing clout to pressure the airlines to install basic safety devices such as better seat belts and oxygen masks or new computer technology proven to reduce runway crashes. Imagine that it was up to the pilots and airline executives whether or not safety measures are taken. Some pilots might want this technology installed on the planes they fly, and they'll go to conferences and get some training on how this technology works, but overall, it's a voluntary ad hoc effort and nowhere near becoming mainstream. Meanwhile, the CEOs of the airlines are preoccupied with trying to keep their companies financially afloat.

The corporate leverage strategy goes only so far because the Fortune 500 companies can exert some muscle on the airlines, but in many geographic areas they may not have the concentrated clout.

This approach begs the question: why should companies that make cars or steel have to work to make another industry—aviation—safe? Why are they the ones doing this? Why isn't the airline industry taking the lead?

Imagine further that some states begin to track how many airline fatalities occur within their boundaries and identify the apparent causes of the crashes. This seems like a sensible thing to do since the information doesn't exist yet. But states have allocated only $20 million in total to track breakdowns in the entire airline industry. And if the plane crashes in a state that hasn't funded any tracking or investigative capacity, families will probably never find out the reason their loved one died.

Imagine that in the meantime, Congress has funded research on aviation safety, and the airlines can use those findings to improve their safety, although no one compels them, and they do so only haphazardly.

At the same time, imagine that the airline industry is fighting efforts by penniless grassroots coalitions of devastated family members whose loved ones died in plane crashes who are trying to establish what we know now as the Federal Aviation Administration, whose mission would be to prevent the 100,000 deaths from airplane crashes every year, and the National Transportation Safety Board, which would investigate airplane crashes.

Meanwhile, the airline industry successfully lobbies Congress to shield itself from the cost of lawsuits when planes crash, and the President signs a bill that caps compensation for survivors' and families' pain and suffering at $250,000. Lawyers are discouraged from taking any cases on behalf of families who have lost loved ones because the contingency fees they would obtain based on economic damages aren't worth their effort. So families cannot recoup any of their economic losses, let alone any other losses.

Imagine further that when crashes occur, no lessons are learned because everyone involved is protecting themselves. It's not known whether they were caused by pilot error, a failure in the equipment, air traffic controller error, the weather, or whatever. The airlines work hard to keep reports of airplane crashes out of the spotlight of the media. Tensions among all the parties obfuscate any effort to find out what really happened. Families never know what caused the crash that killed their beloved.

Would this be a sound strategic plan to reduce deaths from airline crashes? Of course not. So why would we think it a sound strategic plan to reduce medical errors? The fact is *there is no long-term strategic plan to reduce medical errors*. Many dedicated people are working hard to reduce errors. But there's no overall game plan.

In the FAA's most recent federal budget, one of its stated goals is to reduce fatalities from airplane crashes in the United States by 80 percent by 2007. This is a goal of an organization that: 1) is accountable to the public for achieving it, in partnership with the industry and others in aviation; and 2) has the authority to require the airline industry to take actions to achieve the goal.

There is no game plan yet to prevent deaths and serious injuries from medical errors. Without it, they'll keep coming—another million deaths a decade.

Today's Work, Tomorrow's Future

On any night in cities and towns all across America, untold numbers of people from all walks of life are lying awake: a daughter mourning the loss of her mother; a mother wondering about the purpose of life now that her son is gone; a son longing for his father; a father anguishing over the death of his baby daughter; a wife and mother suffering the physical pain of a body grossly ruptured; a doctor despairing over the diagnosis he missed; a nurse fearing that the next mistake will be the one that really harms; a wife missing the warmth of her husband; a husband longing for his wife.

What will tomorrow bring? It is hard to believe that the collective sorrow and pain that is felt at this moment by all who suffer deeply will not emerge, rise, and be a force for change. It is too widespread to be stopped by the wall of silence anymore. The pain has grown so powerful; it can no longer be ignored

Today's work is tomorrow's future. The work ahead may be unpleasant; admitting error and making it known to the public are not easy. Perhaps it is little different from how cancer patients react to the realization that they have to begin a difficult regimen of chemotherapy. Bitter medicine may be the only medicine, but a small price to pay for a brighter future for us all.

14 | Protecting Yourself

When Dr. Mark Chassin, a physician leader known for his work to improve the quality of patient care, was asked whether patients and families should take precautions while in the hospital, he says, "I'm of two minds. Would I recommend it? Absolutely. It can make an important difference to protect against error. On the other hand, it's crazy. Hospitals should be the safest places."

The fact is they are not. But forewarned is forearmed. There are steps that patients and families can take to protect themselves. Among the most notable are the tips from the federal government's Agency for Healthcare Research and Quality (www.ahrq.gov), the agency that is the "point person" on medical errors in the federal government.

Some of the best advice, though, comes from the people you have met who have had the misfortune of firsthand experience watching the health system unravel before their eyes. Here are some steps they recommend:

Know that medical mistakes can happen. You'll remember Ockie, who went into the hospital for cancer surgery but died after a tragic error. His daughter, Rebecca, recalls vividly that, "We never thought for a second about error when we brought our dad to the hospital to have surgery. We were thinking about how we could support him when he got home."

By knowing that mistakes can occur, you can be on the lookout for them. We all know that car accidents happen—we've seen them on the highway, and chances are pretty good that many of us will be involved in an accident at least once in our driving lifetime. But most of us don't think about mistakes in the hospital. Now that word is getting out about medical errors, though, it might be worthwhile to take a page out of the lessons from the defensive driving manual and be alert to the possibility of medical errors. The National Safety Council says that 77 percent of motor vehicle accidents are due to driver error. Of course, the difference with medical errors is that the patient or family isn't in the driver's seat, and sometimes they aren't even in the car when medical errors occur. But even if you're in the back seat when it comes to medical errors, know that they can happen, and that your vigilance can possibly prevent a terrible tragedy.

Know as much about body repair as home repair. Rebecca says that when her dad was originally diagnosed with an aggressive cancer, the family did as much research about the disease as they could, and she recommends that patients and families learn as much as they can about the disease or injury that is affecting them and their treatment options—down to every detail.

A physician who has experienced medical errors as a cancer patient, and who has made errors while practicing medicine, has a unique perspective and says, "It's so important for patients to be informed about their care. They need to know as much about body repair as home repair."

Learn all you can to find the doctor that is best for you. Another seasoned patient suggests that people do thorough research about the doctor who will be performing a procedure or providing treatment. She advises, "Find out as much as you can. Ask people. Find the specialist who does the surgery you need. Just don't go to anyone. You really just need to educate yourself. Get a second opinion. If there had been some place where I could look up my doctor's record, in retrospect, I would have."

Susan, who had the laparoscopic procedure, has the following advice for would-be patients. "Don't put blind trust in doctors. Ask questions and delve deeper. If a doctor says there is a certain risk, don't be satisfied with that. The patient needs to probe and say, 'Tell me more about that.' Don't take everything your doctor says at face value."

Yet another seasoned patient says, "Research your doctor. You can go online. There's the Federation of State Medical Boards Web site, but you have to pay for the information. Then go to the county courthouse. In my county you can find every medical malpractice claim that has been filed in the county—not just the cases that have settled. You can find out all the details. But if the doctor practiced in a different state or county, you probably won't know where so you won't know where to look."

Understand what "board-certified" means. Eighty-nine percent of physicians are board-certified, which means they have been evaluated by their peers through rigorous examination. But read the fine print. Physicians in some specialties who received their certification prior to a certain date might be certified for life and are not required to be recertified.

For example, a physician who is board-certified in ophthalmology who received his or her certification before July 1, 1992, has certification that is valid for life. If a physician certified before July 1992 takes the test and fails, he or she can still retain the title "board-certified." The American Board of Ophthalmology Web site says, "Lifetime certificate holders who fail to pass the renewal process are entitled to retain their lifetime certificates." Ophthalmologists who were board-certified after July 1992 must successfully complete the recertification process every ten years to retain their status.

The American Board of Internal Medicine does not require doctors certified before 1990 to have their knowledge and skills retested. Their certification is for life. Internists certified after 1990 must pass the rigorous examination to retain their board-certified status.

The American Board of Medical Specialties (www.abms.org) can provide information on whether a doctor is board-certified, but you'll have to contact the specialty board to find out the year the physician was certified.

Obtain a copy of your medical records and read them. A New England man wants others to know how important it is to obtain a copy of their medical records and review them. He said, "My wife's death from a misdiagnosed cancer probably saved my life. After she died, I thought I'd better get a copy of my own records since I had the same primary care physician she did. Sure enough, there was an ultrasound report in there that showed I might have cancer, but the primary care physician didn't follow up on it, and neither did the new doctor who took over his practice. It's a good thing I did because it probably saved my life. When I showed it to the doctor, he ordered the follow-up tests that should have been done a while ago, and sure enough, I had cancer. Surgery fixed it and I'm still here to tell about it." He says an added benefit accrues when patients ask to review their medical record, and he uses the exact same words as Susan, who had the laparoscopic procedure: "They take you more seriously."

Keep your own journal. A detailed journal of the care provided can be an indispensable asset. The husband of a Connecticut woman kept such a journal for the more than four hundred days she was hospitalized with a hospital-acquired infection. As mentioned earlier, he recorded every doctor who came to see her, when, and for what purpose. That journal was instrumental in having the hospital settle the case. Lewis's mother, Helen, recommends the same thing: "Write down all procedures, medications, vital signs, and, if possible, fluid intake and output so that someone will have a coherent record."

Trust but verify. This is a good mantra for would-be patients and their families. If you are planning to be in the hospital, especially a teaching hospital, find out who is taking care of you and their role—whether it is a nurse, resident, fellow, or veteran physician.

Don't be afraid to ask. As noted earlier, even the physician-founder of the quality movement in health care, Dr. Avedis Donabedian, couldn't tell who was who on the hospital floors. In sum, know who you are dealing with.

When you are in the hospital, know how to contact your doctor. If you are anticipating a hospital stay, discuss with your doctor—in advance—how he or she can be reached by phone afterward. "Always have your doctor's phone number in your pocket and call him directly if you have concerns," Lewis's mother, Helen, suggests. If he will be away, find out who the backup is.

If you know someone is going to be in the hospital, try to be there "24/7." Family members repeatedly say how important it is to be present in the hospital as much as possible and to watch everything that is done to the patient. If something is going into the mouth or any other part of the body, know what it is and why it has been prescribed, how much has been prescribed, what the effects will be, and how long it is to be taken. When you go home, learn more about the medications on the Internet.

A physician who was undergoing treatment for cancer describes how she witnessed numerous errors in her care. When she had to be hospitalized, she hired a private-duty nurse. She says, "I just wanted someone to be there and watch me. It was the most important thing I did to safeguard my health while in the hospital. There was an office right there in the hospital to arrange for a private duty nurse. In fact, some of the private-duty nurses work at the hospital and do this as moonlighting, which is good because they know the people and how things work. I have told everyone I know who is going into the hospital to get a private-duty nurse." Of course, not everyone can follow this advice because private-duty nurses cost money, and many patients and families can't afford it.

A daughter says how important it was for her family members to take shifts being with their hospitalized father so his basic needs were met. Her brother wrote, "For the first several days my father was there at the hospital, no one bathed him or offered to assist him. The socks that were on his feet when he arrived remained there, unchanged, for three days. One of my brothers traveled from out of state and bathed my father for the first time on the third day of his hospital stay. Because my father was in isolation, his meals were left outside his room, and no one came to feed him other than my family members, who had traveled hundreds of miles to be at his side."

If you hear nothing after a test is conducted, don't assume that everything is okay. Several of the people you've met had diagnostic tests performed, and the reports were sent to their primary care physician. Unfortunately, those reports lingered in their medical records, sometimes for years, yet they contained critical information about progressive diseases the tests had uncovered. Don't assume that the doctor who requested the test has read your report. It may not be his or her fault; it could be the result of one of those administrative snafus, or it may be carelessness and inattention. Call and find out the test results and ask that they be sent to you. Some people may not want to know the results, fearing they might hear the worst. The fact is, if you wait, the medical condition may only worsen.

Follow your gut instinct. If something doesn't seem right, it probably isn't. If you have a nagging doubt, ask. You may have to take matters into your own hands to save your own life or that of your loved one.

For some families, their watchfulness and advocacy made all the difference between life and death. Yet for many others, the best advice on how to avoid harm rings hollow. They watched like hawks at the bedside of their loved one, spoke up repeatedly when things didn't seem right, and did their research. They did everything the experts say you should do, and it still didn't prevent harm. All their love and devotion wasn't enough. Devastating errors still occurred. They ask themselves over and over again whether there was anything else they could have done, and those questions may haunt them for a very long time, if not forever.

One family member puts the advice on how people can protect themselves into perspective. "Patients can't fix this problem. If, as a nurse at the bedside of my mother virtually the entire time in the hospital, *I* couldn't prevent something terrible from happening, we are fooling ourselves to think that patients and their families can do it. I used to say it was important to ensure that a family member is present, but in my case, it didn't work. It might matter in some circumstances, but it's not the answer. It's worth doing that, but I am so afraid that people will be under the illusion that they will be safe. Errors in health care are going to be prevented only if the system does its job."

Notes

Chapter 1

1. Sarah A. Webster, "Hospitals Hide Errors That Kill, Injure Patients: Report Blames Fear of Lawsuits for Health Industry's Silence," *Detroit News*, 6 February, 2000, A1.
2. Kevin Roberg, "Kelsey's Story," *American Journal of Health-System Pharmacists* 58 (2001): 987.
3. Linda T. Kohn, Janet M. Corrigan, and Molla S. Donaldson, eds., for the Committee on Quality of Health Care in America, Institute of Medicine, *To Err Is Human: Building a Safer Health System*. Washington, D.C., National Academy of Sciences, 1999.
4. Troyen A. Brennan, Lucian L. Leape, Nan M. Laird *et al.*, "Incidence of Adverse Events and Negligence in Hospitalized Patients: Results of the Harvard Medical Practice Study I," *New England Journal of Medicine* 324 (1991): 370–376.
5. Karen M. Sandrick, "Raising the Bar," *Trustee*. Online at www.trusteemag.com. Accessed October 30, 2001.
6. Mark R. Chassin, Robert W. Galvin, and the National Roundtable on Health Care Quality, "The Urgent Need to Improve Health Care Quality." *Journal of the American Medical Association* 280 (1998): 1004.

Chapter 3

1. Robert J. Blendon, 2000 International Health Policy Survey of Physicians, The Commonwealth Fund/Harvard School of Public Health/Harris. Internet online at www.cmwf.org. Accessed February 13, 2003.

2. Robert J. Blendon, Catherine M. DesRoches, Mollyann Brodie *et al.*, "Views of Practicing Physicians and the Public on Medical Errors," *New England Journal of Medicine* 347 (2002): 1933–1940.

3. "National Survey on Americans as Health Care Consumers: An Update on the Role of Quality Information." The Henry J. Kaiser Foundation and the Agency for Healthcare Research and Quality. December 2000.

4. Eric J. Thomas, David M. Studdert, Joseph P. Newhouse *et al.*, "Costs of Medical Injuries in Utah and Colorado," *Inquiry* 35 (1999): 260.

Chapter 4

1. Steven H. Miles, *Trustworthy Medicine: The Hippocratic Oath*. New York: Oxford University Press, 2003, in press.

2. *Hippocrates*. Volume VII. Translated by W.D. Smith. Cambridge, Mass.: Harvard University Press, 1994, p. 213.

3. Troyen A. Brennan, Lucian L. Leape, Nan M. Laird *et al.*, "Incidence of Adverse Events and Negligence in Hospitalized Patients: Results of the Harvard Medical Practice Study I," *New England Journal of Medicine* 324 (1991): 375.

4. Lewis Thomas, *The Fragile Species*. New York: Scribner, 1992.

Chapter 5

1. James T. Reason, foreword to *Human Error in Medicine*, edited by Marilyn Sue Bogner. Hillsdale, NJ: Lawrence Erlbaum Associations, 1984.

2. Albert Wu, "A Major Medical Error" Curbside Consultation section, *American Family Physician* 63 (2001): 985.

3. Mark R. Chassin and Elise C. Becher, "The Wrong Patient." *Annals of Internal Medicine* 136 (2002): 826–833.

4. Cited in Lani Luciano, "Reducing Medical Errors and Improving Patient Safety." The National Coalition on Health Care and The Institute for Healthcare Improvement, February 2000, p. 10.

5. Gordon M. Sprenger, "Sharing Responsibility for Patient Safety." *American Journal of Health-System Pharmacists* 58 (2001): 989.

6. J. Brian Sexton, Eric J. Thomas, and Robert L. Helmreich, "Error, Stress, and Teamwork in Medicine and Aviation: Cross-Sectional Surveys," *British Medical Journal* 320 (2000): 745–749.

7. Julie Appleby and Robert David, "Teamwork Used to Be a Money Saver, Now It's a Lifesaver,"*USA Today*, 1 March 2001, p. 1B.

8. Steven R. Daugherty, DeWitt C. Baldwin, and Beverley D. Rowley,

"Learning Satisfaction and Mistreatment During Medical Internship: A Survey of Working Conditions," *Journal of the American Medical Association* 279 (1998): 1195.

9. DeWitt C. Baldwin, Steven R. Daugherty, and Beverley D. Rowley, "Unethical and Unprofessional Conduct Observed by Residents During Their First Year of Training," *Academic Medicine* 73 (1998): 1198.

10. Randy Kennedy, "Residents' Hours Termed Excessive in Hospital Study," *New York Times*, 19 May 1998, p. A1.

Chapter 6

1. Linda H. Aiken, Sean P. Clarke, Douglas M. Sloane *et al.*, "Hospital Nurse Staffing and Patient Mortality, Nurse Burnout, and Job Dissatisfaction," *Journal of the American Medical Association* 288 (2002): 1987–1993.

2. Judy L. Smetzer and Michael R. Cohen, "Lesson from the Denver Medication Error/Criminal Negligence Case: Look Beyond Blaming Individuals," *Hospital Pharmacy* 33 (1998): 640–657.

Chapter 7

1. Mark H. Beers, Michele Storrie, and Genell Lee, "Potential Adverse Drug Interactions in the Emergency Room," *Annals of Internal Medicine* 112 (1990):61–64.

2. Christopher Snowbeck, "Getting It Write: Changing the Low-Tech Way Prescriptions Are Written and Records Are Kept Could Help Reduce Medication Errors," *Pittsburgh Post-Gazette*, 26 June 2001, p. F-1.

3. Richard Knox, "Prescription Errors Tied to Lack of Advice: Pharmacists Skirting Law, Massachusetts Study Finds," *Boston Globe*, 10 February 1999, p. Metro:B1.

4. David W. Bates, "A 40-Year-Old Woman Who Noticed a Medication Error," *Journal of the American Medical Association* 285 (2001): 3134–3140.

5. Stacy A. Wiegman and Michael R. Cohen, "The Patient's Role in Preventing Medication Errors," in *Medication Errors*, ed., Michael R. Cohen. Washington, D.C: American Pharmaceutical Association, 1999, p. 14.3.

6. *Medical Bloopers*™ day-to-day calendar, Salt Lake City: E.P. Publishing, 2001.

7. David W. Bates, Nathan Spell, David J. Cullen *et al.*, "The Costs of

Adverse Drug Events In Hospitalized Patients," *Journal of the American Medical Association* 277 (1995):307–311.

8. Rainu Kaushal, David W. Bates, Christopher Landrigan *et al.*, "Medication Errors and Adverse Drug Events in Pediatric Inpatients," *Journal of the American Medical Association* 285 (2001): 2114–2120.

Chapter 8

1. Steven H. Miles, *Trustworthy Medicine: The Hippocratic Oath*, New York: Oxford University Press, 2003, in press.
2. Marilyn S. Fetter, "Nursing Mistakes: The Institutional Response," *MedSurg Nursing* 10 (2001):58.
3. Jennifer Steinhauer and Ford Fessenden, "Medical Retreads: A Special Report, Doctors Punished by State but Prized At The Hospitals," *New York Times*, 27 March 2001, p. A1.
4. ibid.

Chapter 9

1. Robert J. Blendon, Catherine M. DesRoches, Mollyann Brodie *et al.*, "Views of Practicing Physicians and the Public on Medical Errors," *New England Journal of Medicine* 347 (2002):1933–1940.
2. "Unto the Last," *Four Essays on the First Principles of Political Economy*. New York: John Wiley & Son, 1866. Cited in *Medicine in Quotations: Views of Health and Disease Through the Ages*, eds., Edward J. Huth and T. Jock Murray. Philadelphia: American College of Physicians-American Society of Internal Medicine, 2000, p. 190.
3. Michael J. Berens, "Nursing Mistakes Kill, Injure Thousands," *The Chicago Tribune*, September 10, 2000. (Online at www.chicagotribune.com/news/specials/chi-000910Nursing1,1,1721181.story). Accessed February 23, 2003.

Chapter 10

1. U.S. Department of Commerce, "The Emerging Digital Economy II." Washington, D.C.: Economic Statistics Administration, Office of Policy Development, 1999.
2. Julie Appleby and Robert Davis, "Teamwork Used To Be A Money Saver; Now It's A Lifesaver," *USA Today*, 1 March 2001, p. 1B.
3. Karen Sandrick, "Raising the Bar," *Trustee*, October 2001. Online at www.trusteemag.com.

4. Stephen R. Sleigh, "Health Care Cost and Quality: Prospects for Mutual Gain," *Proceedings of the 54th Annual Meeting of the Industrial Relations Research Association Series.* Atlanta, January 4–6, 2002.

Chapter 11

1. Robert J. Blendon, Catherine M. Des Roches, Mollyann Brodie *et al.*, "Views of Practicing Physicians and the Public on Medical Errors," *New England Journal of Medicine* 347 (2002): 1933–1940.
2. A.B.Witman, D.M. Park, and S.B. Hardin, "How Do Patients Want Physicians To Handle Mistakes?" *Archives of Internal Medicine* 156 (1996): 2565–2569.
3. Steven S. Kraman, "A Risk Management Program Based on Full Disclosure and Trust: Does Everyone Win?" *Comprehensive Therapy* 27 (2001): 257.
4. "Directors to Quit Over Fatal Medical Error," *The Daily Yomiuri*, 17 August 2002, p. 2.

Chapter 12

1. Robert J. Blendon, Catherine DesRoches, Mollyann Brodie *et al.*, "Views of Practicing Physicians and the Public on Medical Errors." *New England Journal of Medicine* 347 (2002): 1933–1940.
2. ibid.
3. Steven S. Kraman. "A Risk Management Program Based on Full Disclosure and Trust: Does Everyone Win?" *Comprehensive Therapy* 27 (2001): 257.

Chapter 13

1. Quoted in Michael Lasalandra, "Harvard Prof Urges Hospitals to Spot, Curb Bad Doctors," *Boston Herald*, 30 March 2001, p. 18.

Index

NASA, 163–165

nasogastric tube anecdote, 18–20

National Practitioner Data Bank
contents, 138–142
privacy of, 153–154

"never events"
keeping score, 223–224
reporting of, 163

New York
practitioner Web site, 151–152
quality initiative, 180
reporting requirements, 162

norms, shifting of, 235–236

nurses
intervention by, 99
perceived value, 113–115
private-duty, 243–244
reasons for leaving, 103–106
skill mismatch, 110
understaffing, 100–102

nursing homes, 44

overtime, 106–107
overwork, 81

Pacific Northwest, 178–179
pecking order, 90–91
peer review failure, 137–138
perforated ulcer anecdote, 31–35
physician orders, 84–85

Pittsburgh, 179–180

polypharmacy, 119

postoperative care, 66–67

prescribing
computerized systems, 172–173
inappropriate drugs, 118–121

priorities, 108–109

private-duty nurses, 243–244

procedures
modification process, 12–13
motivation to change, 55–56

professionals
contact information, 243
emotional support for, 197
experience identification, 233–234
finding one, 240–241
listening skills, 198–199
mistakes on, 204–205
practitioner data bank, 138–142
relationships between, 61–62
reluctance to address problems, 70
suit opinion, 212

public opinion
on quality of care, 49
on suits, 212

quality of care
market pressure, 177–179

ROSEMARY GIBSON is a leader in innovation in health care, making cutting-edge improvements in the care of patients and their families for more than twenty years. She was vice president of the Economic and Social Research Institute and served as senior research associate at the American Enterprise Institute. Ms. Gibson has been a consultant to the Medical College of Virginia and the Virginia State Legislature's Commission on Health Care. She has written books as well as articles that have appeared in the *Wall Street Journal* and the *Journal of the Royal Society of Medicine*.

JANARDAN PRASAD SINGH is an economist at the World Bank. He has been a member of the International Advisory Council for several prime ministers of India. He worked on economic policy at the American Enterprise Institute and on foreign policy at the United Nations. He has written extensively on health care, social policy, and economic development and has been published in many periodicals, including the *Wall Street Journal*.